ATHLETE, NOT FOOD ADDICT

Wellspring's Seven Steps to Weight Loss

Daniel S. Kirschenbaum, PhD, ABPP

New Horizon Press
Far Hills, New Jersey

Copyright © 2014 by Daniel S. Kirschenbaum, PhD, ABPP

All rights reserved. No portion of this book may be reproduced or transmitted in any form whatsoever, including electronic, mechanical or any information storage or retrieval system, except as may be expressly permitted in the 1976 Copyright Act or in writing from the publisher.

Requests for permission should be addressed to:
New Horizon Press
P. O. Box 669
Far Hills, NJ 07931

Daniel S. Kirschenbaum, PhD, ABPP
    Athlete, Not Food Addict: Wellspring's Seven Steps to Weight Loss

Cover design: Charley Nasta
Interior design: Scribe Inc.
Author photo courtesy of kidsinthehouse.com

Library of Congress Control Number: 2013947757

ISBN-13: 978-0-88282-464-2

New Horizon Press

Manufactured in the U. S. A.

18 17 16 15 14   1 2 3 4 5

AUTHOR'S NOTE

This book is based on the author's research, understanding of the science of weight management, clinical work and personal experiences. In order to protect privacy, names have been changed and identifying characteristics have been altered except for contributing experts.

For purposes of simplifying usage, the pronouns him/her and s/he are sometimes used interchangeably. The information contained herein is not meant to be a substitute for professional evaluation and therapy.

DEDICATION

To the 20,000 parents and grandparents who trusted the author
and his colleagues in Wellspring to help their overweight
children, teens and young adults transform their lives.
We have honored that trust and aspired to earn
it every day over these past ten years.

TABLE OF CONTENTS

Part 1: **An Alternative to Food Addiction**

Introduction   3

Chapter 1:   Nurture Your Own Weight Controller-Athlete   9

Part 2: **Understanding Three Things that Can Help Every Weight Controller**

Chapter 2:   Food Addict: An Unfortunate View of Weight Controllers   31

Chapter 3:   Implications for Weight Controller-Athletes   47

Chapter 4:   Becoming Overweight: Causes and Fixes   75

Part 3: **Wellspring's Seven Steps to Become a Weight Controller-Athlete**

Chapter 5:   Step 1—Understand Your Body's Resistance to Weight Loss   93

Chapter 6:   Step 2—Develop a Powerful Commitment to Change   105

Chapter 7:   Step 3—Manage Food to Lose Weight Most Comfortably   113

Chapter 8:	Step 4—Use Movement to Level the Playing Field	157
Chapter 9:	Step 5—Develop an Athlete's Healthy Obsession	173
Chapter 10:	Step 6—Build a Winning Team around You	187
Chapter 11:	Step 7—Become Undisturbable	199

Part 4: **Foodstuffs**

Chapter 12:	Dietary Tips for Following the Wellspring Plan	245
Favorite Wellspring Recipes		253
References		279

PART 1

An Alternative to Food Addiction

Introduction

"My drug of choice is food."
"I'm a compulsive overeater."
"I'm an emotional eater."
"I know I have to accept the fact that I'm a food addict before I can hope to lose weight and keep it off."
"I crave chocolate. I have to have my chocolate fix every day. I know it doesn't make sense because I'm really overweight, but nothing else will do."

Every day in the media and daily life you can hear overweight people talking about the addiction that they believe controls them, an addiction to food. You may be one of them, someone who believes you face overcoming an addiction in order to become a successful weight controller. Some overweight people do indeed face such a challenge. Eating food, particularly certain kinds like sugary foods, can hijack the brain and make weight control difficult, especially for some people. However, that's not the case for the vast majority of overweight people. In this book, you will learn a different concept—one that will empower you to change.

Most weight controllers are not food addicts; they are athletes. Weight controllers face what is essentially an athletic challenge. All athletes must battle the resistance of their bodies to run faster, play harder and get better. In a remarkably similar way to the biological challenges faced by athletes, weight controllers must fight their bodies' resistance to lose weight and keep it off. This perspective on the weight controller-athlete, focused on in this book, can become a truly motivating force for good.

EXAGGERATION ABOUT THE FOOD ADDICT

Unfortunately, the fifty billion dollar diet industry thrives on misinformation, like the idea that all overweight people are food addicts. They spin it out to millions, ensuring confusion and fueling desperation among those seeking slimmer and healthier bodies.

Some Questionable Questions

- Will eight glasses of water help me lose weight?
- Should I take omega 3 fatty acid pills?
- Do cashews make the perfect snack?
- Is there magic in blueberries? Soy? Juicing?
- Will diet sodas kill brain cells?
- Are boot camp trainers the way to slim down?
- Can an ab roller roll away belly fat?
- Is the solution between my ears?
- Low carb?
- Low fat?
- Mediterranean?
- Am I a food addict?

Every day we read and hear in the media that food is a drug. Some claim that food is the "drug of choice" for overweight people and that all overweight people binge eat in order to cope with their emotions. This ostensible addiction causes and maintains obesity and is the toughest of them all. You can give up alcohol or cigarettes or heroin forever, but you have to keep eating, don't you?

In this book I use science to debunk the myth that almost all overweight people can become addicted to food and that addiction causes and maintains obesity. You and I will consider the meaning of addiction applied to weight problems. If you believe that you are a food addict, then that belief may engender a feeling of hopelessness about the possibility of succeeding. After all, this addiction notion implies that you're battling a force more powerful than yourself—a very strong, biologically anchored addiction, a force that controls you. We'll review the substantial evidence that shows that you control your own fate as a weight controller and that it's time to free yourself from the belief that your emotional problems cause your weight problems.

The argument against the food addict myth (for the vast majority of weight controllers) comes from many years of published research, all of which will be summarized clearly. Most definitions of dependence or addiction to a substance require several elements. These elements include the development of tolerance to the effects of the substance and powerful withdrawal symptoms when withdrawing from the substance. Food does not produce these effects. A pint of high-fat ice cream consumed today does not lead to gorging on two pints tomorrow, even among people who identify themselves as "carbohydrate addicts." Research also shows relatively immediate improvements in moods and no withdrawal sickness, as soon as overweight individuals begin a healthy weight-controlling regimen.

We'll also discuss the fact that challenges the food addiction notion most directly. That is, very few obese people binge eat consistently. How can frequent binge eating cause obesity if most obese people do not binge eat? This perspective gains even more traction when realizing that causes other than consuming food compulsively definitely cause weight problems (e.g., genetics; our obesogenic culture; sedentary living).

ATHLETES, NOT FOOD ADDICTS

After challenging the impact of food addiction for most weight controllers, you'll discover the many advantages of considering yourself an athlete, not an addict. First and foremost, you'll learn that losing weight requires you to overcome your body's resistance to losing that weight. You'll read about the five major ways in which your body "thinks" it is protecting you from starvation by making it incredibly difficult to lose the pounds and maintain that weight loss. Then, we'll focus on the parallels between attempts to lose weight and all other athletic challenges. The bodies of athletes resist getting faster, stronger and better. That's why athletes train so hard and so consistently to succeed.

You'll learn more about how athletes succeed by reading about the science of expert performance. This research shows that almost everyone believes that talent helps athletes succeed far more than it actually does. The evidence, you'll be surprised to see, favors one of baseball great Willie Mays' favorite sayings: "The harder I work, the luckier I get."

Some examples from the research on expert performance will, I believe, help convince you of the power of learning versus inherited talent. You might expect most child prodigies to become expert performers as adults. These children can play piano or golf (or do other remarkable things) at incredibly high levels when most other children still struggle to tie their shoes. Yet, the research shows that most of these prodigies do not become experts as adults. Also, the vast majority of expert adult performers were never prodigies as children. Many expert musicians, for example, show early interest in music, but they become experts by getting instruction early in their lives, practicing a great deal and gradually developing exceptional skill.

Expert performance research also documents the amazing adaptability of the human body. The number of capillaries supplying blood to muscle cells changes after a few weeks of training. Muscle fibers can change from fast twitch to slow twitch and vice versa, depending on practice levels. Fast twitch muscles facilitate bursts of speed while slow twitch muscles maximize endurance. Changes in lung capacity, bone density, heart size and aerobic capacity occur when training increases. Researchers have even found that differences in the percentages of slow twitch fibers in athletes' muscles occur only for muscles specifically trained for their sports. For example, the legs in runners and back muscles in kayakers show these changes, but arm muscles do not change in these athletes in parallel fashion.

The body's adaptability and the limited impact of inherited talent help encourage working hard to develop new skills. The research also underlines that point by showing the value of deliberate practice in many different sports and domains of performance. That is, elite performers consistently differ from their non-elite peers in the amount and intensity of their deliberate practice. For example, runners at the national level train on average 4.9 times per week; runners at the regional and local levels train 4.2 and 3.2 times, respectively. Outcomes of marathon races can be predicted very accurately from knowing the regularity and amount of practice during the nine weeks prior to the race.

To lose weight, you will have to work pretty hard, but you do not have to become an athlete in the usual sense of the term. You do not have to train for a marathon or compete in any sport to lose weight and keep it off. You have to become a weight controller-athlete. You can do this first by thoroughly understanding your body's resistance to weight loss. Then, you can use the athletic concept to develop an athlete's mindset that takes your physical and mental game to new levels. Those athletic steps will fuel your power as a weight controller, allowing you to succeed most comfortably and effectively.

CHAPTER 1

Nurture Your Own Weight Controller-Athlete

Athletes harness enormous power to smash tennis balls over 130 miles per hour, to run sub-five minute miles for twenty-six miles in a row and to dominate opponents on all fields of play. The best of them use something better than practice to do it: they use perfect practice. That includes great understanding of the physical demands of their sports, excellent instruction, support from teammates and coaches and remarkable mental games. Weight controllers can benefit from parallel elements to develop their own versions of sustainable weight-controlling power.

This book uses as its roadmap or training guide *The Wellspring Weight Loss Plan,* an approach my colleagues and I have developed for the world's most successful network of therapeutic weight loss camps for overweight young people and adults. Wellspring is the leading provider of weight loss services for overweight young people in North America. You will learn about the key elements of the food plan used within Wellspring. The Wellspring Plan serves as the basis of the programs provided by Wellspring over the past ten years. Wellspring focuses its treatment on immersion programs, an approach that involves twenty-four/seven participation in nearly ideal weight-controlling environments (camps, boarding schools and residential programs) for extended periods of time. Two books and more than two dozen articles in peer-reviewed scientific journals have documented the remarkable effectiveness of Wellspring's programs, as have numerous documentaries and segments on most major TV magazine shows, feature stories in many magazines and virtually every major newspaper in the US.

The real-life success stories which I describe next bring these objective findings to life. Wellspring has documented hundreds of remarkable transformations. Let's look at some amazing success stories. Then I will present some of the more objective evidence to illustrate the value of this approach.

Letters from a Father about his Son's and Family's Remarkable 3.5 Year Weight Loss Journey: Dave and Stevie M.

12/5/13
Dear Wellspring,
It has been three and a half years since Stevie attended camp. I want to share his pictures with you. When Stevie arrived at camp he was twelve years old, 5'4.5" tall and weighed 187.6 pounds. He lost 19.4 pounds in four weeks at Wellspring Pennsylvania. Today, he is sixteen and stands 6"1" and weighs 160 pounds. I don't normally take the time to do stuff like this, especially three years later when most people may not remember Stevie. But, I thought it was important.

A few years ago, Stevie was the "fat kid" that no one wanted on their team; other kids would make fun of him on the ice during hockey and he was the slowest kid on the baseball team. That has all changed.

Please let everyone at Wellspring know that if they are ever having a bad day, or question why they are working for Wellspring, to take a look at this picture, or read my letter. The work they are doing is so important that they need to know how they have changed his life. He has improved at all the sports he played. He played travel baseball last year and is still in hockey. He was the fourth leading scorer on his team last year and scored more goals last year than all of his other years combined. He is also continuing his baseball and has become one of the best hitters. He is still on plan, he eats well and never strays. He has incredible willpower, even when temptation surrounds him.

I want to thank all of you from the bottom of my heart. Wellspring was worth everything I paid and then some, and I would not hesitate to recommend it to anyone. I would do it all over again, but fortunately I do not have to.

Sincerely,
Dave M

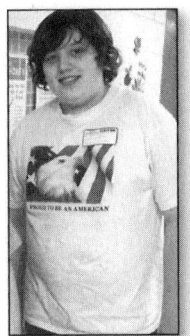 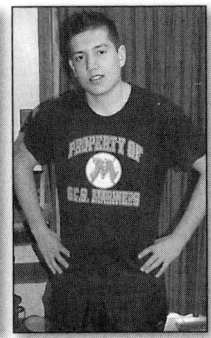 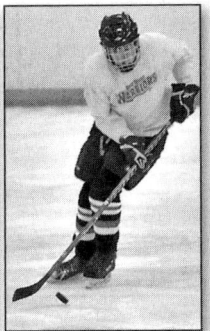 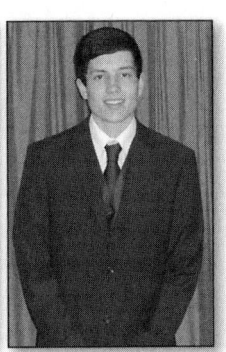

12/5/13
Dear Dave,
Thanks so much for sharing the wonderful news about Stevie, and the great photos, with us. We're hoping that you might be willing to say even more about what your family did to support him so remarkably well over these past 3.5 years.

Thanks again,
Dan Kirschenbaum

12/11/13
Dear Dan,
Sure. I can say a great deal about Stevie's progress and our family's support of him over these past several years.

Stevie was always a heavy kid. I did not think that his diet was all that unhealthy; however, he continued to gain weight as he got older. We became very concerned that he was approaching a very unhealthy size. I was also worried about his potential lifespan carrying that much weight and about the seemingly free pass people get for making fun of the fat kid. Even though he had lots of friends, you can always hear the mockery from the outside.

My wife and I obviously did not have the tools needed to help him and made the decision to do something about it. I did a lot of research on weight loss camps for children and decided on Wellspring after careful consideration.

My main concern was that Stevie would be starved for four weeks and then run like a dog. He'd then lose a bunch of weight at camp, only to put it back on when he returned home. So I was really worried after we dropped him off at Wellspring Pennsylvania for his four weeks of camp.

On his first call home, I only had two questions for him. Are you ever hungry and are they making you exercise too much? He told me that he was never hungry and that there was always enough food to eat. That made me very happy and helped to allay some of my fears. He also told me that he loved all of the activities. Even though he was heavy, he always liked sports and activity was not the problem. I have to say that he really liked and admired Hidi, the fitness coach. He had a very positive influence on Stevie. Stevie still talks about his floor hockey experience playing against Hidi. Since he was the only kid that had ever played hockey, he quickly became the star player in floor hockey. That was a huge boost to his confidence.

My wife and I both attended the family workshop weekend at the end of camp. I will say that it should be mandatory, because the parents have just as much to do with the success with the program as the child does. It was very eye opening. I did get the opportunity to sit down at lunch and dinner with the president/co-founder of Wellspring (you!) and was able to ask a lot of questions. I appreciated your time and insight.

We also met with Stevie's Behavioral Coach who told us that if any child would be successful going home, it would be Stevie. I had concerns about why Stevie would eat so much and was worried that he might be depressed or have some other emotional issue. His BC told me that Stevie was very well adjusted and ate because he was hungry, plain and simple. That means that his weight problem had more to do with what we fed him—and his particular genes/biological tendency to gain weight easily.

The ride home from camp was tough. We were not prepared very well for the trip. The snacks we had for the ride were not on plan. So it was basically submarine sandwiches and apples. When we finally got home, we had to empty all of our cupboards and the fridge. We stocked up on non-fat and extremely low-fat products. It takes time to re-write your menu, but we had all of the recipe books that Wellspring provided and used that as our baseline. We tried just about everything to see what we liked best. You had a slogan at the training that was something like this: "Find lovable foods that love you back." That is basically what we have lived by since coming home from camp.

The day after we got home, Stevie had a team baseball party at our house. This was very important to him. He was torn because Wellspring made an offer to extend his stay two more weeks and he had such a great time and made some great friends. However, he gave up being on the all-star team in baseball to go to Wellspring and this party meant a lot to him. We took the advice from Wellspring that "kids will eat healthy if that is what is presented to them." We had melon, watermelon, fat-free brownies, fat-free rice crispy treats, fat-free hot dogs, salad with fat-free dressing for the team party on the day after we returned from camp. This was another big boost for Stevie. His friends and coaches were amazed at the transformation and the food was all eaten with no complaints; so Stevie did not have to feel like he was different.

We found a local bison farm and we buy bison meat for hamburgers, which is even leaner than lean beef. We always have fresh fruit, yogurt, gelatin and other "free foods" around to eat. There has not been a high-fat cookie, cake or anything of that sort in our house for three and a half years. Any desserts we have are homemade cakes or treats from the recipe book Wellspring provided. We also purchased some low-fat cookbooks to help out. Unfortunately, I have a sweet tooth, but I will not bring any junk into the house for Stevie's sake. So it has to be homemade.

Obviously we have the issue with Stevie visiting friends and spending the night. We would go over the plan with his friends' parents and sometimes send food with Stevie that he could eat just to be sure he is not hungry. We have some very good friends who really supported him and accommodated him while he would visit. Most people know at this point that he only eats healthy very low-fat foods. Our friends and family make mistakes sometimes, but they mean well. I try to explain it like this to people: imagine you had Celiac disease and you could not eat gluten. Those people have to change their diet or die. We treat fat for Stevie like gluten. We have to eliminate it. He cannot eat it. It is his gluten. I hope that makes sense. Obviously there is some fat in the diet. Even vegetarians must find it hard to avoid it at some level. And, the word "moderation" is not in our vocabulary. Moderation doesn't work. It takes a healthy obsession to beat this problem. That is something that many people do not understand.

At this point, we really don't do much for Stevie. Our shopping habits have been modified; we know what to buy; we know what is good to eat. So it is pretty easy. My wife and I also eat the same way as Stevie and both of us have lost a lot of weight. We are not as good as Stevie because he has a mental log of everything he eats and really does not crave junk food. He is amazing! He likes low-fat smoothies; he loves fruit. He has changed. It is a big commitment. Healthy food costs more; fresh fruit and veggies can add up, but we and Stevie know what the alternative is. So, we all want to do what is right for his heath—and ours.

To give you an idea of how this affected his life, he had an assignment at school that required him to put together pictures of himself and make an historical collage. He was procrastinating on the project and really would not work on it. The teacher contacted us and told us he was not making progress. My wife talked to him about it and he told her that he did not want to put pictures of himself pre-Wellspring for people to see. That was the old Stevie and he is the new, improved Stevie and he doesn't ever want to be seen or known as the old Stevie. So we really did not know how important it was for him to be thin and healthy. He was given another assignment instead.

I think, in general, friends and family understand his struggle. They will ask us what they should make, what can he have? You cannot run away from it; you have to say, I am sorry, I cannot eat that. Then you can ask, "Do you have something else I might have?"

We do not eat out much anymore unless we are traveling. Lunch is usually [a sub shop] and for dinner, we try to find a Mongolian BBQ, which is awesome for Stevie. Everything is healthy. You can build your dinner online and get the calories and fat before you make your meal, but most of it is veggies; so it is all free food so he can eat well and not be hungry. We also will review menus online for local restaurants where we will be visiting and make our decisions on where to eat based on the healthiness of the menu. We also have found a local pizzeria that has fat-free cheese. That is a life saver, because every once and a while, you gotta have pizza. In fact, if we have guests, we won't even tell them it is fat free and no one knows the difference.

We also have Mongolian BBQ night at home: we cut up all different veggies, shrimp, chicken, squash, onions, you name it, then everyone fills their bowl with veggies and shimp and chicken and we have a large griddle, you pick your favorite seasoning, soy sauce or teriyaki, salt, pepper, garlic, all fat free, and then throw it on the griddle just like at the restaurant. It is a huge hit. You ought to try it at camp. Stevie's hockey team loves it.

Those are some of the things we have done. Parents just have to change, too.

I am doing this because I think you have a wonderful program and your people are great. You saved Stevie's life. What more can I say? Sorry if my thoughts are a little scattered, but it's an emotional thing to write about and I am very passionate about it. Thanks again for all you have done.

Sincerely,
Dave M

Finding a Passion for Wellness through Wellspring: Tricia H's Seven Year Journey

Growing up, I was a normal-sized girl with a little bit of a tummy. Throughout elementary and middle school I was somewhat active and played soccer, tennis and golf. But things changed when I turned sixteen and I started boarding school and that is when I began to gain weight. I was not as active as I had been in middle school and I had access to a variety of fattening foods both on and off campus. I ate when I was bored or sad.

By the end of my sophomore year my parents were concerned about my weight. My mother approached me with the idea of my attending Wellspring New York, an all-girls fitness/weight-loss camp, that summer. I liked the idea and began my first summer in 2006 at Wellspring New York for the full eight weeks.

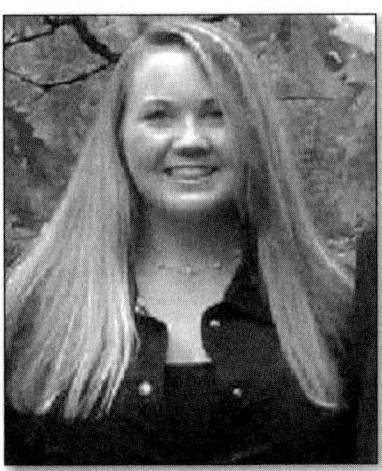
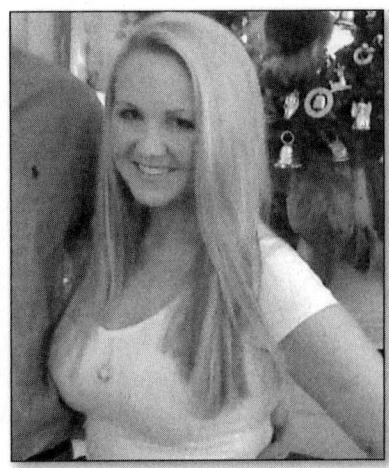

My life changed that summer. I found a passion for fitness classes, jogging and a community that supported and encouraged my weight loss. I learned to manage the foods I loved and shift them into healthier low-fat versions, which further contributed to my weight loss. That first summer, I lost twenty pounds, reshaped my body and my mindset through exercise and classes and transformed my life. While I had gotten my weight down from 194 to 174, I still had more to lose in order to be a healthy weight for my age, size and frame. I continued jogging when I got back to school and made running a part of my daily routine. I lost another ten pounds my junior year at school and the summer before my senior year I decided to return to Wellspring to get off the last 10 to 15 pounds I wanted to lose. Starting my senior year I was down to 150 and felt great. I have maintained a weight between 140 and 150 for the last six years and Wellspring has changed my life.

What is really significant is that for the last five summers I have returned to Wellspring to work as a counselor at Wellspring camps in New York, Pennsylvania and Wisconsin. I am now a certified personal trainer and have taught Pilates and fitness classes for three of the five summers. I have helped Dr. Kirschenbaum with parent workshops by speaking about the program and how it has worked for me. I am immensely grateful for this program and to have been given the opportunity to attend Wellspring and transform my life.

Katya F's Healthy Obsession: Four Years and Counting

January 23, 2009 is the day I picked up my first self-monitoring journal (or SMJ), strapped on my first pedometer and started using the Wellspring approach to change my life. It was my first day at Wellspring Academy [Wellspring's former year-round boarding school in California] where I learned how to become a successful, long-term weight controller living my own version of a healthy obsession. The result of this is that I lost a whole person (130 pounds) over the course of a year and have kept it off.

Early on, it was extremely apparent that living the "Wellspring Plan" was far beyond any time frame or goal to lose a specified amount of weight. It was a lifestyle change that took an extremely simple approach (but not an easy one). I learned how to implement it into my daily routine. Experiencing the plan with this mindset allowed me to develop my daily focus on planning what I would

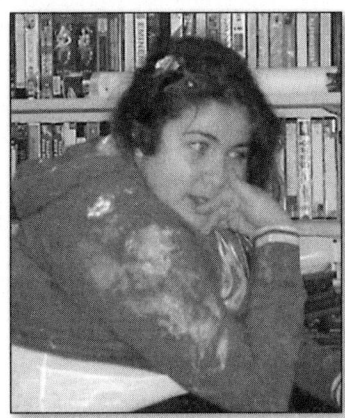
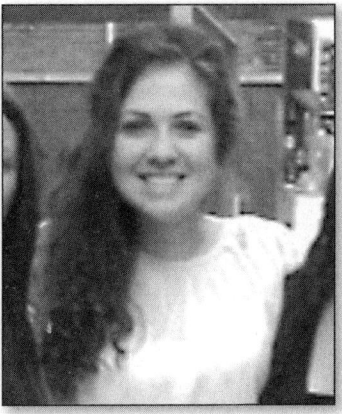

eat and how I'd get my activity up to a very good level. Eventually, it became like brushing my teeth on a daily basis.

As a result, I feel healthy and in control. Ten thousand steps a day went from being a goal to a requirement. Self-monitoring my food and being aware of fat intake became second nature.

Every now and then, lapses have occurred. While they do not happen frequently, because of my planning and dedication, combined with a fear of gaining my weight back, I continue to remind myself to stay in control. I stayed on plan using the basics that I started to learn on January 23, 2009. I have been truly blessed with a great opportunity to attend Wellspring and learn about what a healthy obsession is and create my own.

A Letter from Brendan R's Mom: From a Critically Sick Baby to a Motivational Marvel

My son Brendan attended Wellspring Wisconsin during the summer of 2012. He was an obese seventeen-year-old. He was 5'10" and 248 pounds. I want to share his amazing journey because I am so thankful for the Wellspring program and so proud of Brendan's accomplishments!

Brendan was born with a life-threatening birth defect—Biliary Atresia. Only one in 15,000 babies are born with it, and without a liver transplant he would have died. After seven months of waiting, he received his life-saving liver transplant two weeks before his first birthday. This yellow, skinny, sickly baby transformed into a pudgy, healthy, beautiful child. But as he grew up he became more and more

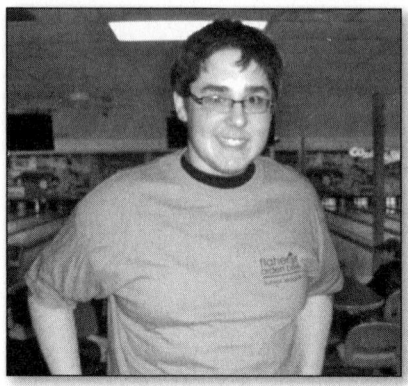 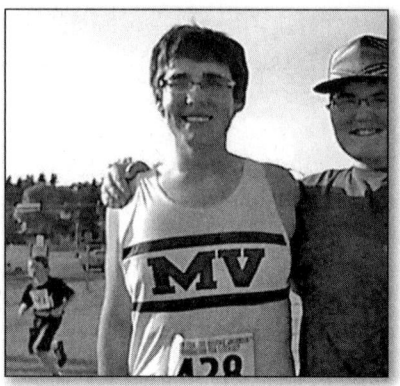

overweight, and I guess I just didn't care because he was alive and we were just so thankful to have him. But to see his struggles with acceptance and low self-esteem as he became a middle schooler and on to high school, I decided that maybe it was time to get serious about his weight issues.

I had a lot of unhealthy food around the house and didn't even know it because I rarely read labels except the front of the boxes. We ate out a couple times a week because life is just hectic when you're a single mom raising two kids. One night watching TV we found "Too Fat for Fifteen: Fighting Back" on the Style Network [a TV series based at one of Wellspring's boarding schools] and were fascinated watching these kids struggle with their weight and do so well getting healthy. I read the stories on the website and was a bit skeptical. How could six weeks at a summer camp change my child's life when all my encouragement over the last seventeen years didn't change anything? Plus we'd tried dieticians, health clubs, low-carb diets…and nothing worked. Well, little did I know that this camp would be one of the best things to ever happen to Brendan and this entire family!

Brendan's first few weeks at camp were tough. His weekly call consisted of tears and begging me to come and get him. And as the mom of a once critically-ill child I was tempted to cave and go get him. But I didn't. When I came to camp for Family Weekend three weeks later, I was shocked when two of his counselors told me he was an "ideal camper." Seriously? My overweight, video game-playing kid was participating? And losing weight? And when Brendan saw me, he gave me a hug and said he would stay and finish at camp and was starting to have fun. And by the end of camp he was made Team Captain of the Wellspring games!

At Family Weekend, I learned so much valuable information! I was floored that losing weight didn't mean eating bland, boring food. I went home, cleaned out all the cupboards of all the fattening foods, and started cooking Wellspring recipes and inventing my own. I began eating the Wellspring way too. I lost ten pounds and am now a size six. Brendan, after six weeks at camp, lost thirty-seven pounds and continued losing another thirty-one pounds since coming home. He has maintained his weight now for nine months at 180-185 pounds (5'10"). What he learned at Wellspring is his healthy obsession. He reads labels on almost everything he puts in his mouth. If he does gain a little weight, he cuts back on his food intake or goes out for a run.

Speaking of running, Brendan was not active before Wellspring. He played a little baseball his freshman and sophomore years of high school (in an all-abilities league) and had a lot of fun, but he was overweight, slow and lacked confidence on the field. He won two awards: Most Improved and "Most fun to watch steal second base—all three minutes of it." Funny, but sad. But that was the old Brendan. The new Brendan joined the cross country team at school! He ran and ran and enjoyed it and made new friends. His best time for running a 5K was 32.26 minutes. His coach nicknamed him Slim. Slim! Can you believe it? He continues to run and lift weights. His healthy obsession now is to stay in shape and keep his weight at or below 185 pounds. Friends and family are absolutely amazed when they see him and the transformation he has made.

Some of our favorite foods we make at home are pizza (low-fat frozen pizza dough and marinara sauce, fat-free hot dogs, vegetables and fat-free cheese) and anything on white rice. Spray butter and fat-free chicken broth are used to cook most of our food; if we want a treat I buy the lowest fat brownie mix I can find and use fat-free yogurt and egg beaters instead of oil and eggs and I bake them in mini muffin tins and keep them in the freezer. I make pancakes (always use a nonstick pan so you use no fat) with fruit and sugar-free syrup. We buy low-fat, flavored protein powder and blend with frozen fruit. I can't keep enough bananas and grapes in the house as that's about all Brendan snacks on—except pretzels and mustard for dipping. We plan ahead when we aren't home by bringing fat-free yogurt, fruit, rice cakes, tuna or chicken salad sandwiches made with fat-free mayo and spices.

> Brendan's cross country coach wrote this in his graduation card: "Brendan, you are the essence of persistence: The race goes not always to the swift but to those who keep running. You have powers you never dreamed of. You are capable of doing things you never thought possible. There are no limitations on what you can do. You have an inspirational story to tell. You had a dream and you worked extremely hard to reach your goals. I am very proud of the young man that you have become."
>
> I am so thankful for this amazing program at Wellspring. You and your staff have changed Brendan's life in ways that never would have happened if he hadn't attended camp.
>
> — Jill R.

Chloe S: A Bodybuilding Champion Just Two Years After Camp

Chloe began camp in 2011 and weighed 185 pounds at that time. Two years later, she weighs 75 pounds less and has become a figure competitor champion (a class of bodybuilding). Here's how her mother, Jen, raved about the change and Wellspring's role in it:

> None of Chloe's recent success could have been realized without the help (and jumpstart) that Wellspring Camps gave her! Not only were the eating habits and activities that were taught invaluable, but the emotional support was priceless! Chloe realized, after only six weeks at Wellspring, that she could achieve ANYTHNG that she wanted to if she put her heart and mind to the task! Wellspring was the best investment I ever made for Chloe.
>
> — Jen R.

I asked Chloe to describe how she related to this process, from the time she and her parents considered the Wellspring idea to the present. Chloe mentioned that she was reluctant to go to Wellspring, but that she was tired of the verbal bullying she experienced. She also wanted to fit in with her friends better and to have guys be attracted to her more than they seemed to be at the time.

Chloe's mom, Jen, thought that the timing was good too. Chloe was a sophomore in high school at the time she agreed to go to Wellspring and had already tried Weight Watchers and many other diets. Something always seemed to "get in the way of Chloe's success."

Jen mentioned that Wellspring's approach seemed so much better than the others she tried. She didn't feel tired at all, as she had on the

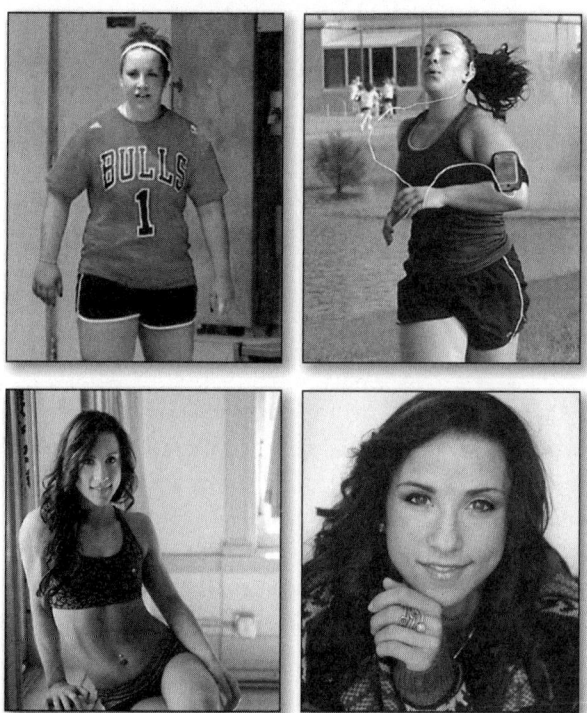

Ann Latinovitch Photography

Atkins diet. She liked that the *Wellspring Plan* is a way of life, not a diet. She also loved the momentum she created by losing 25 pounds in the six weeks at camp vs. the 10 pounds she lost on the Atkins diet in three months. Chloe also emphasized that she found that the other campers and staff members really motivated her, through their accomplishments, role modeling and emotional support.

Chloe keep careful track of her eating and activities after camp. She used a fitness tracking app on her smartphone to do so and reported that she never exceeded the Wellspring maximum of 20g of fat per day. She also started running almost every day. She found a highly motivating trainer and met a successful body builder. Chloe found that she really liked the weightlifting and body building quest. She nurtured the healthy obsession she developed at camp and now clearly uses that healthy obsession enthusiastically every day.

Chloe also acknowledged the strong support she received from her mother. Jen made Chloe's food completely in accord with Wellspring's very low fat approach, plus Jen continued her favorite role: as Chloe's most dedicated cheerleader.

OBJECTIVE EVIDENCE ABOUT THE WELLSPRING PLAN

These inspiring stories only hint at the scientific value of the Wellspring approach. Case studies add humanity to science, but they do not show systematic effects based on thorough and controlled research. My colleagues and I created Wellspring based on scientific evidence, but also based on an emphasis on keeping the approach simple (easy to understand and remember, but not easy) and sustainable. Still, creating a program based on science does not show the degree to which it actually works when brought to life in the real world. The research evidence does, however, lend some objective balance to the heart-warming qualities of the hundreds of success stories that have emerged from Wellspring's programs.

In the first published paper that reviewed all published articles in professional journals focused on immersion treatment, my colleague, psychologist Kristina Pecora Kelly, and I found something remarkable. When we summarized the results of twenty-two studies in that publication, we discovered that those programs that combined immersion (twenty-four/seven care for at least ten days) with cognitive-behavioral therapy (CBT) produced results that seemed far better in the long run compared to results typically obtained in high-quality outpatient programs. CBT is an approach to helping people master problems in living by relying on principles from psychological and biological sciences. It includes an emphasis on problem solving, goal setting, self-monitoring (observing and writing down relevant information) and stress management. CBT serves as the core element to assist in the process of changing lifestyle behaviors that we use in Wellspring.

Figure 1-1 illustrates that discovery. Specifically, it shows reductions in weight (measured in percent overweight) to be almost 200 percent better in immersion programs with CBT than in programs that didn't include CBT or outpatient CBT programs. Wellspring and one other group, researchers led by Dr. Caroline Braet from the Zeepreventorium in Belgium, have published studies that account for these outstanding results.

Figure 1-2 shows the results recently published based on follow-ups completed at Wellspring's camps. Note that, on average, campers continued to lose weight even after they went home, just like the five young people in the case studies presented previously in the introduction. Here's the bottom line: Wellspring's approach has

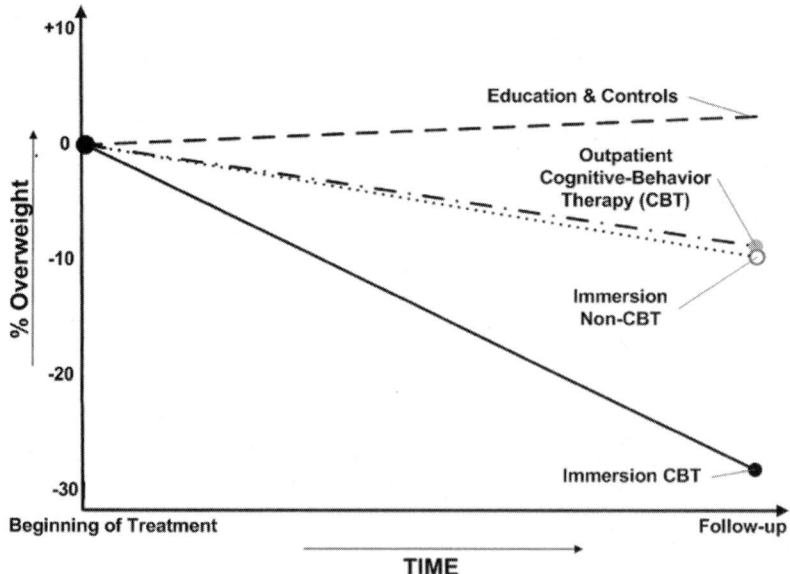

Figure 1-1. Change in percent overweight comparing education/controls, outpatient cognitive-behavioral therapy (CBT), immersion without CBT and immersion CBT. Graph based on Kelly and Kirschenbaum (2011) and reprinted with permission.

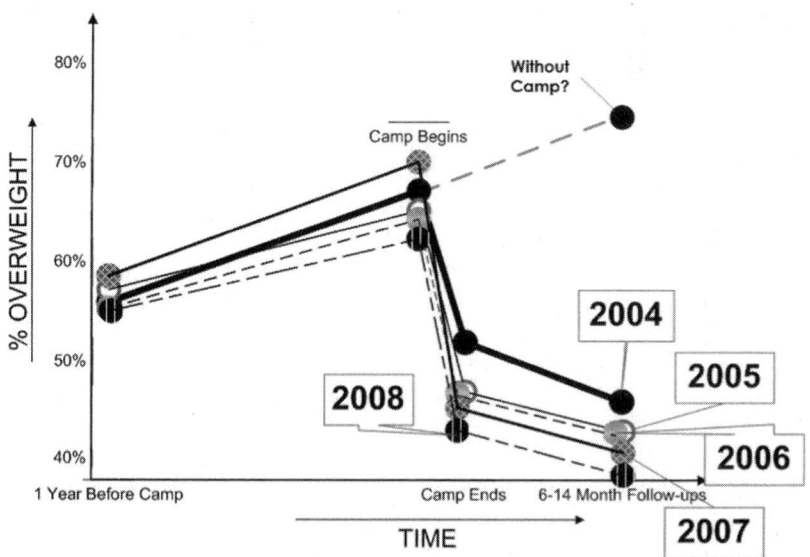

Figure 1-2. Change in percent overweight for Wellspring campers from one year prior to camp through six to fourteen month follow-ups (2004-2008).

produced among the best outcomes ever reported for any treatment of weight problems.

Wellspring's programs rely on the following seven steps to help its clients nurture and maximize their own weight controller-athletes. You'll first read more about the myth of food addicts, the weight controller-athlete concept and then the causes of weight problems and how to fix them. Then, you will find a full description of each of these steps.

1. Understanding the Biological Resistance to Weight Loss

More than a dozen powerful biological forces combine to resist permanent weight loss. These include the permanence of excess numbers of fat cells. Overweight and formerly overweight people have billions of fat cells that shrink, but don't die, when people lose weight. Each cell can increase volume by twenty thousand fold. Never-overweight people have about one third to one sixth as many of these cells. Unfortunately, in their shrunken states following weight loss, these fat cells act as hungry baby sparrows with their mouths chronically open looking for more fat.

The dozen biological resistances to weight loss come from our genetic ancestors—hunter-gatherers from two hundred thousand years ago. At that time, and for almost all of the past two hundred thousand years, natural selection would have promoted great efficiency in fat storage, and resistance to weight loss, as survival mechanisms.

However, biology is *not* destiny. Just as all athletes learn to overcome their biological resistances to get stronger, faster and better, so, too, can weight controllers learn to manage their biological challenges.

2. Creating a Powerful Commitment to Change

3. Managing Food to Lose Weight Most Comfortably

Eight principles of eating that keep food fun and keep appetite quiet (higher numbers indicate the most critical elements; 1 to 10 scale of importance, with 1 = minimally important to 10 = vitally important, critical):

- Very Low Fat = 10
- Calorie Consciousness = 9
- Low Caloric Density = 9
- Eat Your Calories, Don't Drink Them = 8

- Find Lovable Foods That Love You Back = 8
- Protein Power = 6
- Avoid Sugary Snacks = 5
- High Fiber = 3

4. Using Movement to Level the Playing Field

We'll consider the many advantages of maintaining an active lifestyle, including using a pedometer every day and targeting 12,000 steps per day. The advantages of high levels of activity include:

- Expends more energy (helps create the negative energy balance necessary for weight loss)
- Increases metabolic rate
- Promotes use of fat consumed for immediate energy, rather than storing the fat for later use in the fat cells
- Improves commitment
- Improves mood
- Improves sleep

5. Developing an Athlete's Healthy Obsession

Consistent self-monitoring creates a greater awareness of long-term goals, improves coping with stressful situations and greatly enhances weight control. Successful athletes focus a great deal of their attention on their training regimens. They plan their days around them and make sure they get the coaching and support required for success. Masters of weight control do the same things. We'll review the scientific evidence that supports these points, including an important study conducted at the University of Florida that showed that weight controllers who pursued the goal of exercising every day far outperformed those who targeted three to four times per week over time. Studies of highly successful weight controllers also support this definition of a healthy obsession: *A healthy obsession is a sustained preoccupation with the planning and execution of target behaviors to reach a healthy goal.*

6. Creating a Supportive Team

Structure works for long-term success. Part of that structure could include a support group (like a TOPS group—Take Off Pounds Successfully) and certainly includes support from friends and family. This chapter reviews how to obtain and maximize such support.

Imagine the plight of a competitive swimmer who had minimal access to a pool or a ski jumper who lived in Florida. Weight controllers who can modify the foods in their home cupboards and the kinds of meals prepared do far better than those whose environments include constant challenges. Environments can facilitate healthful eating and consistently high levels of activities, or they can create challenges at every turn. The chapter on this step will review methods for creating supportive environments that you can use to increase your weight-controlling power.

7. Becoming Undisturbable

Lapses can become relapses, injuries can cause early retirement and daily hassles and other stressors can weaken self-regulatory strength. Ten primary stressors and ten keys to stress management will be presented in this chapter. In brief, anticipating high-risk situations armed with a variety of powerful coping skills can help weight controllers manage the inevitable setbacks without becoming derailed. You *can* become undisturbable.

ABOUT YOUR COACH—
THE AUTHOR

I have had the privilege of helping thousands of people become successful weight controller-athletes. I've refined and tested this approach in clinics at the University of Cincinnati, University of Rochester, University of Wisconsin, Northwestern University Medical School and in my own clinic in Chicago (the Center for Behavioral Medicine and Sport Psychology) and in Wellspring over the last forty years. I've also published eleven other books and more than one hundred and fifty articles in peer-reviewed scientific journals.

One of my books, *The Treatment of Childhood and Adolescent Obesity*, was the first one published to help professional therapists assist overweight young people; one of my more recent books, *The 9 Truths about Weight Loss*, was unanimously endorsed by the American Council on Exercise as "the best book ever written for the public on how to lose weight and keep it off." Over the past ten years, I helped develop Wellspring, which has grown to become the leading provider of treatment services for overweight young people in North America. At its heart lies the concept featured in this book: the weight controller is an athlete, not an addict.

I've used this approach myself, transforming myself from a kid who was nicknamed "Chubsy" when he was eight years old and a teenager who was thirty pounds overweight to become a healthy and active weight controller-athlete for more than forty years.

PART 2

Understanding Three Things that Can Help Every Weight Controller

CHAPTER 2

Food Addict: An Unfortunate View of Weight Controllers

On many popular TV talk shows, food addicts are discussed and viewed as the primary explanation for obesity. According to this theory, people gain excess weight because they are food addicts. They use food as their drug of choice. If you struggle to control your weight, this food-drug supposedly helps you to get through the stresses and strains of everyday life and it most certainly helps you to manage major challenges. For you as a weight controller, think of what this characterization says about you.

It says:

- If you struggle to lose weight, you binge eat every day and you are an addict.
- If you fail to lose weight, you are an addict.
- If you succeed at losing weight, you are a food addict now in recovery.
- If you have a weight problem, you are dependent on binge eating to get you through each day.

Do those notions seem to fit you? I've worked with thousands of weight controllers over the past forty years. Many of them did, indeed, believe in this addictive notion to explain their weight problems. For a few of them, it actually helped them understand the power of the biological forces that were dead set against their success. For almost all of them, however, their beliefs in the food addiction explanation certainly did not make it accurate. Such beliefs probably made it harder for them to succeed in the long run.

It gets worse the more you think of the implications of those points. The most famous treatments of addictions rely on a twelve-step approach. This approach began in the 1930s and now, more than two hundred self-help organizations, with millions of dedicated followers, use it as their foundation. It's part of our cultural landscape.

Most people recognize its key principles. Those principles create some rather troubling implications for weight controllers. The most disturbing of these suggests that to recover you must recognize that you cannot control this problem. It controls you. And, if you cannot accept that reality 100 percent, you will never recover from its grasp. Does food control you? Millions of successful weight controllers would never agree that it does. Few of them would have ever contemplated that notion on more than a superficial level, let alone use that admission to begin their transformation to slimmer, healthier selves.

Other elements of these core principles would make many weight controllers squirm. The twelve steps say that you can only succeed by realizing that only a higher power can provide you with the strength to succeed. These steps also require you to admit that you harmed others due to your addiction and that you must make amends for those errors. That requires acknowledging to others that your addiction to food somehow harmed them and then you're supposed to ask for their forgiveness.

Did your eating really harm others? The causes of excess weight reviewed in chapter 4 indicate that most obese people do not eat that differently from non-obese people. If this is true, than how could your style of eating cause so much damage to others? Do you have to rely on some unseen force to change your lifestyle? Successful weight controllers succeed by relying on lots of movement, very low-fat diets, the support of others and focusing consistently on their goals.

These introductory points raise major concerns about viewing weight controllers as food addicts. However, this viewpoint has gained tremendous traction in recent years. Food addiction recovery groups now exist and endorsements of this view flood all forms of media with increasing frequency. Let's take a closer look at the concept, the evidence used to support it and the problems with it.

FOOD ADDICTIONS AND FOOD ADDICTS: DEFINITIONS

Some researchers argue that the dramatic increases in obesity throughout the world correspond to increasing availability of cheap, high-fat and high-sugar foods. Could it be that people become addicted to such foods—and this powerful force has caused epidemic increases in obesity? Some parallels do exist between the brain chemistry associated with drug addiction and the effects observed (especially in animals) after consuming a lot of sugar. This is particularly true for the way certain nerve cells in the brain release the chemical dopamine and the effects on various sites in the brain that follow.

Some parallels observed in pleasure centers in the brain between drugs known to cause addiction and the intake of high doses of sugar, by itself, make a very weak case for the usefulness of the food addiction notion for most weight controllers. Other forms of fun and excitement also produce related changes in brain chemistry. Are we addicted to engrossing movies or funny stories or exciting sales in department stores? In order to meet a reasonable standard for addiction, researchers have argued that other criteria deserve consideration.

For example, Gearhart and Corbin (2012) compared food addiction to a widely recognized set of criteria used to define "substance dependence." They relied on a document compiled via consensus from many professionals and used every day to determine insurance reimbursement and to diagnose psychological problems, *The Diagnostic and Statistical Manual for Mental Disorders* (DSM). The term *dependence* has become generally preferred to addiction in professional circles because it's a broader concept and less reliant on strictly physical effects of a substance. Dependence is sometimes used as a synonym for addiction and these terms are considered to reflect a greater degree of severity than substance abuse. Dependence also focuses on the more observable aspects of a person's behavior to define a major substance abuse problem.

DSM defines substance dependence as the presence of at least three of seven diagnostic criteria over the past twelve months; in addition, *the person must show a serious degree of distress or impairment in functioning* in order to qualify as someone with a dependence problem. In addition to the distress/impairment caveat, the seven other criteria are listed on the next page. After reviewing them, let's consider the degree to which overweight people are typically affected by serious distress and the other criteria of addiction.

1. Tolerance (physiological) to increasing amounts of the substance
2. Withdrawal effects when use of the substance is discontinued
3. Loss of control
4. Repeated failed attempts to reduce or stop consumption
5. Substantial time spent to obtain, use and recover from use of the substance
6. Giving up important activities
7. Continued use despite physical or psychological problems

Serious Distress or Impairment

This caveat creates the first problem for believing that obesity results from food addiction. A great many overweight people do not view their weight status as a problem, nor are they impaired by it. Cross-cultural studies demonstrate this particularly well. Among people from Puerto Rico, researchers found that their participants rated photographs depicting obese individuals (on the mild side of the obesity spectrum) as very attractive. Certainly many significantly overweight people work, maintain families and do not show evidence of serious distress or impairment. My colleagues and I found that overweight people who sought professional help showed more distress than those who had similar weight problems but did not seek help. The latter group, in our study of employees at a major hospital, reported the usual level of stresses and strains of everyday life, no more or less.

Many researchers have documented related evidence. A great many obese children and adults function very well and do not show evidence of psychological distress or significant impairment. For example, Shelly Greenfield and Michele Crisafulli recently reported dramatically elevated levels of psychological distress among those who have substance use addictive disorders (SUDs) compared to population norms. They reported that about 30 percent of those with SUDs had mood disorders at some point in their lives compared to 8 percent in the general population. Greenfield and Crisafulli also noted dramatically higher rates (three to twenty times higher) than normal among SUDs for a variety of other serious psychological disorders. These included anxiety disorders, psychotic disorders and personality disorders. In sharp contrast to people with SUDs, most studies show either no difference in psychological functioning or mild elevations of such problems among obese individuals. In our own research at Wellspring, for example, the average score on a general measure of psychological distress that we've obtained repeatedly for thousands of Wellspring campers has hovered right at the population average.

The people in your own life will show these patterns, too. Think about the many overweight people you know or have known. How many of them seemed to function quite well in their lives, at least compared to other people who did not have weight problems? Sure, about 10 to 15 percent of people struggle with serious psychological issues and many seek help for these problems. But does weight status determine who seeks such help or not? In contrast, think of those you know who struggled with alcohol or other addictive substances. If you know people who have had such addictive disorders, you probably also know that a high percentage of them had problems with their moods, anxieties, relationships and personalities.

Tolerance

Tolerance means that the person needs increasing amounts of the substance in order to produce the desired effects. People who become dependent on alcohol and heroin, for example, use more and more of these substances over time in order to get high. People do not demonstrate tolerance toward food. If you eat a half pint of high-fat ice cream today and enjoy it, you can eat the other half next month and get the same enjoyment from it. No evidence from scientific studies published to date can refute this point.

Withdrawal

In Wellspring's programs over the past ten years, we have not seen a single case of physical symptoms of withdrawal among the ten thousand participants in all of our programs over that period of time. Both teenagers and adults in these programs radically change their diets (and activities) from the first day they immerse themselves in one of our camps. Yet, none of them have reported flu-like symptoms or raging headaches or seen pink elephants just because they switched to a very low-fat, low-calorie diet. Actually, they generally report feeling better physically almost immediately. None of the researchers who contributed to the recent book edited by Brownell and Gold, all of whom clearly favor the notion of food addiction, could find any evidence to support the existence of physical withdrawal from certain foods.

Loss of Control

Some obese people do, indeed, report binge eating. That usually means eating large quantities of food and feeling a loss of control when doing so. The big question for this criterion concerns the frequency of such binge eating among people who develop obesity. Those who believe that overweight people are best characterized as food addicts would have to argue that almost all obese people frequently lose control of their eating. That's just not consistent with the scientific evidence.

Food addiction advocates might expect that young obese people who participate in one of Wellspring's camps, a controlled setting that prevents binge eating, might exhibit considerable distress. After all, if they binge eat consistently to reduce distress, how could they handle the sudden removal of this ostensibly critical coping device without feeling miserable? What if you played guitar every day and that made you feel good. Then, you lost your guitar. Imagine how you would feel. At loose ends, anxious, frustrated, sad? Thaxton (1982) found that requiring very consistent runners to stop running for a day made them quite distressed. Yet, in our research at Wellspring, and in most studies of cognitive-behavioral treatment of adolescent obesity, overweight teens consistently feel much better as they participate in such programs. The loss of binge eating (for the relatively few who binge regularly) failed to cause the misery predicted by those who believe in food addiction. These robust findings indicate, once again, that binge eating, as a means of coping with distress, probably did not cause people's weight problems.

Repeated Failed Attempts to Reduce or Stop Consumption

In June 2013, Golfer Phil Mickelson came in second for the sixth time at the US Open. He found the most recent near miss in Ardmore, Pennsylvania, incredibly disappointing. Mickelson didn't get out of bed for several days after that sixth silver medal. Yet, just a month later, he flew across the ocean and competed in the Scottish Open. Then, in the following week, the forty-three-year-old played at the oldest and most revered of all major championships in golf, the British Open. He had never won a tournament on such a links course (minimal trees, near the ocean, lots of wind), although he had attempted to win the British Open nineteen previous times. Was his attempt at winning this incredibly important tournament an indicator of a golf addiction? After all, he repeatedly failed (nineteen repetitions) in his attempts to win. After he won both of those tournaments in the span of eleven amazing days, including a final round that was nothing less than spectacular at the British Open, not one commentator or pundit labeled him as an addict or dependent or any other pathologically oriented term. They just admired his skill, talent and persistence and appreciated the new title conferred on all British Open champions: Champion Golfer of the Year.

Those who demonstrate other criteria for substance use dependence or addiction share this quality of persistence with Phil Mickelson and probably all other successful athletes. The best baseball players who ever lived, for example, failed to get a hit more than once every three or so at-bats statistically. Even very successful weight controllers usually fail to lose the weight and keep it off during their first major effort. For cigarette smokers, frequent attempts to quit predict long-term success. If you do not try to master difficult problems repeatedly, especially ones with strong physiological effects, you will not succeed. I believe that including this criterion among the seven just does not make sense.

Substantial Time Spent to Obtain, Use or Recover from Use of the Substance

It does not take much time to buy or smoke cigarettes, yet cigarette smokers are clearly dependent on the use of cigarettes, including a powerful physiological dependence. Similarly, high-fat foods do not require much effort to buy and consume, nor do they require any recovery after use. Consumption of high-fat, high-calorie foods does not meet this criterion, but neither does the use of other addictive substances like cigarettes or caffeine. As in the prior example of repeated failures to succeed, this criterion also does not do well at determining dependence.

Giving Up Important Activities

Alcoholics and heroin addicts invariably become preoccupied with their addictions, including abandonment of jobs and relationships in order to maintain their habits. Weight controllers also avoid certain high-risk situations sometimes in order to maintain control. Such restraint hardly seems to justify a designation of dependence (addiction) on food. On the other hand, some of the relatively few obese people with severe binge eating disorders also avoid others in order to continue their binges or to recover from binges. (A later section of this chapter, Food Addicts by the Numbers, describes the data on which this conclusion is based in more detail.) In view of the infrequency of severe binge eating disorder among obese people, this criterion also fails to support the notion of food addiction.

Continued Use Despite Physical or Psychological Problems

People with common substance use dependences often continue using despite major legal, financial, interpersonal and health problems. Some obese people certainly do continue consuming high-fat, high-calorie foods despite increasing problems resulting from their obesity. However, many use such health problems to motivate themselves to seek treatment, too. Unfortunately, after failing to succeed using a variety of methods, a type of learned helplessness and lack of optimism about success probably contributes to sustained consumption of problematic foods. Why attribute such eating to an addiction versus a lack of self-confidence (sometimes called self-efficacy)?

Conclusion

Table 2-1 summarizes the evidence comparing drug to food addiction on the distressed caveat and the seven criteria used to define substance dependence. The evidence and logic just do not support the usefulness of thinking about the causes of obesity as a food addiction or defining most obese people as food addicts.

EMOTIONAL EATING

Food certainly does not meet the usual standard definition of an addictive substance. Another notion closely allied to the food addict is the *emotional eater*. Of the thousands of overweight and obese people I have known over the past forty years, most believed that they overate because of emotional issues. That perception comes from living in a culture that endorses the food addict concept. This perception also involves making a very common mistake in thinking known in psychology as "the fundamental attributional bias." We tend to attribute causes to ourselves. That bias downplays the importance of biological factors and social/environmental influences.

Table 2-1

Drug Addicts versus Obese People Compared on the Eight Elements of the Diagnosis of Substance Use Dependence (Addiction)

	Drug Addicts	Obese People
Distressed	Very Frequently	Sometimes
Tolerance	Yes, in most cases	No
Withdrawal	Yes, in most cases	No
Loss of Control	Yes	Infrequently
Repeated Failures to Change	Yes	Yes, but isn't persistence at difficult tasks good?
Substantial Time to Obtain	Usually	No
Giving up Activities	Yes, frequently	Rarely
Sustained Use Despite Problems	Yes	Yes, but necessary for survival

Certainly we all get some satisfaction and comfort from eating, at least some of the time. That's not abnormal; it's just human and an important and fun part of being human. It's time to start thinking of yourself in new terms. Eating for emotional reasons does a lousy job of explaining the reasons you have a weight problem. Many better explanations exist, as you will see in the following chapters. The science of obesity does not support emotional eating as a primary cause of obesity any more than it supports the myth of the food addict. The next section puts an exclamation point on that fact.

FOOD ADDICTS: BY THE NUMBERS

Four researchers for The National Institutes of Health published one of the most important papers ever to address the issue of binge eating and made their findings available free on the Internet to anyone interested, even though the study was published in a medical journal, *Biological Psychiatry*. James Hudson, Eva Hiripi, Harrison Pope and Ronald Kessler received substantial grants from a host of federal and private agencies to conduct a comprehensive survey of Americans that measured how many adults ever experienced consistent and excessive binge eating, known as Binge Eating Disorder. These researchers conducted a nationwide series of in-person interviews on 2,980 adults using a standardized and valid structured interview. These adults came from all over the United States and were considered to be a representative sample of adults of all ages.

The researchers asked these adults if they ever met the diagnostic standards for Binge Eating Disorder. According to the standard diagnostic criteria (DSM-IV), they would have defined this disorder as including at least six months of regular binge eating episodes in which the person experienced a loss of control and psychological distress because of the binge eating. However, the researchers used a less stringent criteria requiring only three months of such episodes to qualify for the diagnosis.

Earlier in this chapter, I indicated that those who believe overweight people are food addicts and expect the vast majority of them, maybe all of them, to meet the definition used in this important survey for Binge Eating Disorder are wrong. The survey results dramatically and emphatically show that did not happen.

Figure 2-1 shows that about 69 percent of adults in the US today are either overweight or obese. The survey revealed that only 2.8 percent of adults report any lifetime incidence of Binge Eating Disorder, meaning having any history of substantial amounts of binge eating over a period of three months or more.

Figure 2-2 illustrates these results in terms of numbers of people. We have over three hundred million people in the United States today, of which 74.5 percent are adults. Of the adult group of over two hundred million adults, about 69 percent are overweight or obese (about one hundred and sixty million). Let's say that even one hundred million of those people with weight problems could have been expected to have had substantial trouble with binge eating, at least according to those who believe in the food addict explanation for obesity.

The survey showed far fewer numbers actually reported any problems with binge eating at any point in their lives. Some of those binge eaters were not overweight or obese. Based on the report, 2.8 percent of the total number of adults equals 6.6 million people. Even if the vast majority of those 6.6 million people were overweight or obese, that would mean that only five to six million reported this problem. Figure 2-2 contrasts the 100 million expected by the food addict advocates versus the six million observed via objective research.

Quite a stark contrast, isn't it?

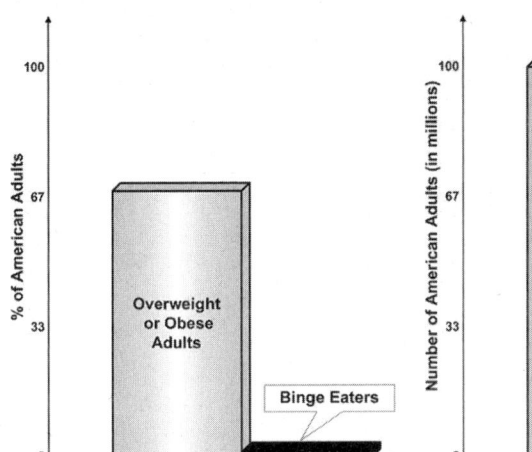 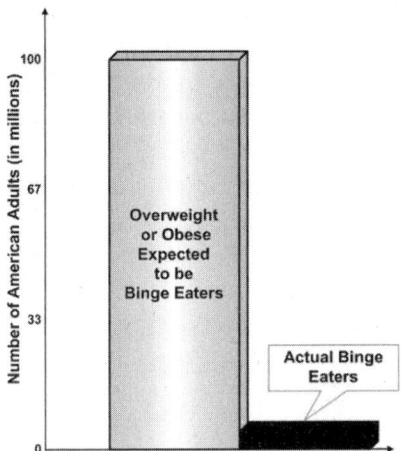

Figure 2-1. Percentage of American Adults Who are Overweight or Obese versus percentage Who were Diagnosed with Binge Eating Disorder in the Survey by Hudson et al. (2007).

Figure 2-2. Estimated number of American adults who would be expected to be diagnosed with Binge Eating Disorder based on the food addict model versus those who were actually diagnosed as such in the survey by Hudson et al. (2007).

Question: Do people identified as "food addicts" in research studies struggle more than others to succeed at losing weight?

Answer: No!

Some scientists believe that addiction to food explains why most people do not lose weight successfully. These addiction advocates also believe that those who suffer most from this addiction would struggle far more than others to lose weight. Consider the clear logic of this. According to the definition of addiction, food addicts, compared to other overweight people, supposedly experience much more distress and hopelessness, binge eat very often, require increasing amounts of food and more binge eating over time, experience withdrawal symptoms when they reduce consumption, and fail repeatedly in their attempts to lose weight. Therefore, food addict believers would predict that overweight food addicts would fail to lose weight much more so than non-addicts.

Two very recent studies tested this prediction directly. Dr. Jacob Burmeister and his colleagues from Bowling Green State University evaluated fifty-seven obese adults using the Yale Food Addiction Scale (YFAS). This scale asks people to indicate the degree to which they experience distress, hopelessness, interference with other aspects of their lives, binge eating beyond their control, withdrawal and related aspects of the definition of binge eating. If participants acknowledge experiencing several of these symptoms quite often, then researchers consider them to be food addicts. The adults studied by the Bowling Green researchers attempted to lose weight for seven weeks. YFSA scores did not predict outcomes any better than a simple measure of binge eating. In other words, binge eaters did not lose as much weight as non-binge eaters in this small study, but the YFAS scores revealed nothing more than that. Binge eating alone is far less of an intractable problem than an addiction and could be changed by simple changes in diet, activity and support for most people.

Some of the best and most prolific researchers in the world who specialize in studying obesity, Dr. Tom Wadden from the University of Pennsylvania, Dr. Gary Foster from Temple University and their colleagues, received substantial funding from the National Institutes of Health to study this issue. Compared to the Burmeister study, Dr. Wadden and his colleagues studied a much larger sample of overweight and obese adults (178) over a much longer period of time (six months). They determined that 15 percent of those adults met the YFAS definition of food addict. Based on their support for the food addiction concept, they expected their "food addicts" to struggle more than the non-addicts to stay involved in the program and lose weight. That did not happen. The food addicts attended just as many sessions and lost just as much weight as the non-addicts.

Various factors could explain these results, but the findings from both of these studies suggest that self-reported food addiction does not disrupt weight management. If food addiction does not affect weight loss, then why continue to use the concept, at least as it relates to the vast majority of weight controllers?

Maybe the Yale Food Addiction Scale just identifies people who strongly believe they eat for emotional reasons. After all, many overweight people and talk show hosts believe that emotional distress causes weight problems more than anything else. They may not understand the powerful influence of other factors that cause weight gain, like genetics, sedentary living and eating too much fat. Many of the thousands of participants in Wellspring's programs and in my clinics would have considered themselves food addicts according to that Yale scale. Yet, when they learned an effective way to lose weight and began thinking of themselves as weight controller-athletes, they started to realize that food did not enslave them. They, and you, have the power to change, especially if you say goodbye to the belief that you're addicted to food.

EXPERT OPINIONS

Some researchers have devoted substantial parts of their careers to understanding the degree to which addictive notions apply to obesity. Editors of two books included articles by many of these devoted scientists. In the oldest of these two volumes, neither the editors, Walker Poston III and C. Keith Haddock, nor any of their many contributors came to the conclusion that obese people are best characterized as food addicts. Dr. Haddock and Dr. Poston summarized the research in their book, *Food as a Drug*, by concluding that foods that we eat generally do not have mood-altering effects that resemble drugs at all:

> *Several conclusions can be made regarding the pharmacological [drug] properties of foods. First, the US government is reticent to label foods, dietary substances or herbs as drugs despite potential medicinal properties of these substances. Second, the food substances that have demonstrated medicinal qualities are either not typically consumed in [high enough] quantities to produce a significant pharmacological [drug-like] effect in the typical American diet unless they are taken via supplementation. Finally, the whole foods typically consumed in the American diet generally have not been found to have significant psychopharmacological [drug-like] or addictive properties (p.143).*

Kelly Brownell and Mark Gold published an even larger and more ambitious book, *Food and Addictions*. Dr. Brownell is a psychologist and among the most widely admired experts on obesity in the world. Dr. Gold is a research psychiatrist, highly regarded as an expert on addictions. Based on my personal conversations with them and knowledge of their writing and research, it has become clear they both view food addiction as a viable and potentially important concept. In particular, they asserted in their book that consumption of high-sugar foods may essentially "hijack the brain and override will." However, even these impressive scientists had to conclude: "Relatively small numbers of people might merit the label 'food addict...'" and, that interventions for these relatively small numbers of food addicts "...can be seen as helping those in need but not having a public health impact on large populations." (p. 439) They also acknowledged that science cannot as yet assert that other types of foods, like the most problematic kind—high-fat foods—can impact people in an addictive fashion.

THE HARMFUL CONSEQUENCES OF VIEWING OVERWEIGHT PEOPLE AS FOOD ADDICTS

On August 20, 2013, British reporter Deni Kirkova described online an unpublished survey of 5,139 members of Slimming World. This organization resembles Weight Watchers in that it includes online and group support to promote weight loss. Here's how Kirkova described the results:

- "Cravings for food can be as bad as drugs: Food addicts get high after their 'hit'."
- 76 percent of the "Slimmers" compared "their weakness to an addict's desire for cigarettes, drinks or drugs."
- 55 percent believed that they got "a buzz" from their favorite high-fat foods in the past.
- 77 percent felt an initial improvement in mood after eating high-fat foods, but 83 percent felt worse afterwards.

Many overweight people, just like these "Slimmers," view themselves as weak, neurotic addicts. Those perceptions do not make the notion of food addict more accurate, by any means. They just show how pervasive this unfortunate view has become.

Such descriptions might also provide a face-saving rationalization. If you were a boxer and lost a fight to an amazingly easy opponent, you would feel awful. What if your opponent was incredibly powerful, a world-class champion? You would probably feel okay about such a loss. Well, if you have struggled to lose weight and keep it off, you might be tempted to view your opponent as unbeatable. Then you would not feel so bad about losing that fight. Viewing food as addictive may ease the pain of the struggle for many in this way: I have not succeeded at losing weight because food creates a powerful, unbeatable addiction. If I do not view food in this addictive way, then I must accept my own limitations or weaknesses (or lack of knowledge about how to lose weight successfully). That does not make the notion more accurate, just more understandable.

Imagine believing this about yourself: I'm a food addict. Do you feel encouraged or empowered? Or do you feel discouraged or helpless? Most people report discouragement. After all, we have all grown up with the twelve-step view of addictions, which begins by the addict admitting very directly to powerlessness: I cannot control this. Also, admitted addicts are negatively tainted by the public's very disparaging view of those with mental disorders. According to studies of these perceptions, people describe individuals with psychological problems as dangerous, unpredictable and even "worthless."

RESEARCH SUGGESTS THE HARMFUL EFFECTS OF THE FOOD ADDICT MYTH

In addition to the negative stigma associated with those with mental disorders, the food addict notion creates far more problems than it's worth. Several lines of research support this conclusion.

Medical Model vs. Social Learning Model

Amerigo Farina and Jeffery Fisher and their colleagues, researchers at the University of Connecticut, taught undergraduates in Abnormal Psychology courses from one of two perspectives. The *medical model* approach asserts that it's best to view problems in life as symptoms of underlying disorders. Diagnosing these disorders is supposed to enable therapists to match treatments effectively to the various types of disorders. The food addict notion fits well with this approach, viewing food addicts as diagnosed patients with additional underlying mental problems. An alternative view, the *social learning model*, asserts that problems in living often occur because people learn maladaptive ways of handling challenges. As such, they can unlearn those patterns and change by setting new goals, problem solving and taking action. In the University of Connecticut research, the participants who received the social learning messages actually viewed change more optimistically and worked on their own issues more consistently during the course. This means that the approach that orients people to the more medical/disease concepts, like the food addict perspective, can decrease active efforts to change.

Optimism Beats Pessimism

Viewing weight problems as caused by an addiction can lead to substantial pessimism about the prospect of changing. That's an inherent part of the definition of dependence: its intractable nature. If you view yourself as a food addict, you view food as controlling you, not vice versa. Your effort to control this problem can feel like a mountain you cannot climb.

Psychologists Michael Scheier and Charles Carver defined what they termed dispositional optimism as the global expectation that good things will be plentiful in the future and bad things scarce. Christopher Peterson summarized the research on dispositional optimism. He noted that optimism affects self-regulation when people face impediments to achieving their goals. In the face of difficulties, do people nonetheless believe that goals can be achieved? If so, they are optimistic; if not, they are pessimistic. Optimism leads to continued efforts to attain the goal, whereas pessimism leads to giving up. Studies on optimism viewed in this way showed that relatively optimistic people tend to feel happier and to engage challenges in more active and effective ways. If the food addict idea breeds pessimism, then it also leads to sadder moods and more difficulties with the process of changing lifestyles.

Resilience Involves Control

You undoubtedly know some people who seem to flourish when faced with life's challenges. That's the basis of the old maxim: when the going gets tough, the tough get going. Certainly coaches want athletes who can handle pressure; not just handle it but excel in the face of it. Michael Jordan always wanted the ball so he could take those shots with seconds remaining and the game on the line. You can bet he viewed himself as a great athlete, not someone who feels out of control, powerless and neurotic.

Psychologist Suzanne Kobasa's research indicates that having control and perceiving something as controllable can help people cope with life's challenges. If you believe you can control your fate, you will seek out ways to take charge of problems. Those who view themselves as food addicts would have trouble doing this; after all, the food supposedly controls them.

CONCLUSIONS

You clearly have a choice: accept a view of yourself as a food addict or find something better. The food addict concept can bring with it pessimism, sadness, a medical model orientation and a less-than-resilient approach to solving the inevitable problems associated with a quest for change. It's time to consider something better: the concept of the weight controller-athlete.

CHAPTER 3

Implications for Weight Controller-Athletes

Think for a few moments about one common element that all athletes share. Compare the challenge of a bowler trying to throw three strikes in a row (a "turkey") to a tennis player attempting to hit a serve to within inches of her target to a runner attempting to run a personal best time. Each of these athletic challenges requires taming the body's resistance to perform. Just because you want to bowl that turkey doesn't mean your body will cooperate. The bowler must learn techniques that promote the release of the ball in a very particular way to a certain board on the lane with tremendous consistency. The tennis player has to master the skills of tossing the ball to a certain height and in the proper position and then moving the racket to contact the ball at exactly the right moment, with an appropriate twist of the wrist and arm. The runner will only reach that personal best if he puts in the time to run many other miles in training, in addition to doing some shorter distances at higher speeds. In each case, these athletes can only achieve their goals by training their bodies to do things all of our bodies naturally resist. It takes time, instruction, mental toughness and other steps to change our bodies' natural tendencies. Those natural tendencies would have us throw bowling balls into gutters, hit tennis balls into the net and run at far less than optimal speed. Athletes must work even harder and longer and better than other dedicated peers.

In this book I stress that weight controllers function much like athletes. We must learn to tame our biological resistances, too. That biological management takes a different direction from athletic performance toward sustained weight loss. Still, athletes train to make their bodies bend to their wills—and so do weight controllers. Next we'll discuss what athletes do to become great at their sports. As you read, I'll point out the parallels.

Let's first consider the highest level of performance—peak performance—and what it takes to accomplish that. Then, we'll look at the process of building such athletic skills. All through this chapter, we'll view the parallels between weight controllers and athletes.

PEAK PERFORMANCE

Athletic feats at the highest level are described as "peak performances." Peak experiences are feelings of joy associated with great achievement. "Flow" is similar to peak experience. It is a very enjoyable state that occurs when performing a task extremely well. People are in flow states when they are automatically meeting the challenges of the task at hand. "In the zone" and "flow" are synonymous.

Sometimes athletes perform exceptionally well, even when they are struggling with some aspects of their games. They somehow manage to scrape together superb performances, despite mechanical or technical flaws. Other times, flow and peak experiences can occur without producing great performances. Tiger Woods, the fourteen-time major champion and seventy-nine time tour winner, understands these points and commented about them in a recent magazine article: "You ask Nicklaus how many majors he won when he hit the ball well all week. He'll say zero. That's what I'm doing. I'm scoring well. I'm not making any big numbers. I'm always in the hole."

Most sport participants relish their flow and peak experiences. They want to know how to achieve these states more often. These are, after all, the ultimate payoffs for hard work and concentration. This chapter focuses on the skills needed to create flow, peak experiences

---

Weight Controller–Athlete Parallel #1:
BIOLOGICAL RESISTANCE
- Athletes overcome biological resistance to peak performance through training and focusing.
- Weight controllers overcome biological resistance to sustain weight loss through their own form of training and focusing.

and peak performances. Before describing elements of practice schedules and other foundations of these experiences, let's consider the nature of peak experiences in more detail.

CHARACTERISTICS OF PEAK EXPERIENCES IN SPORTS

Consider for a few minutes the characteristics of your peak sports experiences. Remember that these are gratifying experiences that usually accompany superior performances. Complete Exercise 3-1 to help analyze the characteristics of your peak experiences. In the exercise, two of my clients are discussed, Renee (a distance runner) and Gary (a competitive amateur golfer). Notice the differences in feeling states associated with the best and worst performances reported by Gary and Renee. The best performances felt easy and produced very positive feelings in each athlete. Renee also reported a special sense of awareness during her unusually good run. Gary reported an unusual degree of confidence when chipping on the last four holes of one of his better rounds of golf.

Studies on thousands of athletes at different levels conducted by Tara Scanlan, Kenneth Ravizza and other researchers have shown that the experiences reported by these two athletes are often part of peak experiences. The anxiety, hopelessness and general unhappiness described in Renee and Gary's worst performances contrast sharply with seven characteristics that define peak experiences:

- effortless and automatic
- acutely aware
- relaxed
- controlled
- very positive and confident, inspired
- fearless
- joyful

Let's consider each of these characteristics so that you can formulate an emerging goal for your weight control program.

Effortless and Automatic

Kenneth Ravizza emphasized that during these peak performances these athletes surrender themselves to the experience. They function as if they "could continue moving forever, no longer having to exert [themselves] consciously."

Exercise 3-1: Characteristics of Peak Experiences in Sports

Try to recall your best and worst sports experiences. Try to identify how you felt in every way during your most satisfying and gratifying moments as an athlete. Outline in the following section the characteristics of that experience. What were you thinking about, how did you feel and what were you aware of during your most satisfying experiences? After completing this section of the exercise, provide an outline of your worst experiences in sports. Again, consider what you were thinking about, what you felt and what you were aware of during those situations. After completing these outlines, think about the main points that occur to you when comparing your best and worst performances.

Performance Descriptions

Description of my feelings during my best performances:

_____
_____
_____
_____

Description of my feelings during my worst performances:

_____
_____
_____
_____

Renee's and Gary's Descriptions of Best and Worst Performances

BEST PERFORMANCES

Renee: One of my best performances was a "turkey trot" around Thanksgiving when I ran my personal best in a 10K. I ran it in under fifty minutes for the first time (forty-nine minutes, eight seconds). More important than the time was the feeling. That run seemed very easy, yet I seemed aware of everything going on within my body and around me! I could feel my feet coming off the pavement at every step. Yet, through a lot of the race my legs felt like they belonged to someone else. They felt powerful and rubbery. I was able to tune in to the other runners around me. I noticed that some looked like they were working very hard. Others were more like me, kind of gliding along.

Gary: Certainly the first time I broke eighty was one of my best performances. This happened about ten years ago. Yet, I still remember it remarkably well. I was playing a familiar course on a beautiful summer day. I knew that if I finished the last four holes in two over par that I would break eighty for the first time. I became aware of this on the fifteenth tee. I managed to finish the last four holes in even par and shot a seventy-seven. The amazing thing is that I didn't land on any of the greens in regulation. I chipped to within three feet or less on all four of those holes. Any golfer can tell you that chipping that close to the pin four times in a row doesn't happen every day. I remember focusing very directly on each of those chips. I felt confident in my ability to get the ball close to the pin on every one of those shots. I also remember feeling a bit tense while I was walking the fairways of those holes. Yet, my tension changed to a very tuned-in concentration when I got to the point of hitting the chips.

WORST PERFORMANCES

Renee: I ran a 5K not long ago that was a real struggle. I felt tired before I started the race. I don't think I was deprived of sleep but nevertheless I felt a bit worn out. I had been training pretty hard in the previous couple of weeks prior to the race. I may have overdone it. It just seemed like a struggle to get through the race in a lousy time. Seemed like everyone else was just blasting past me while I huffed and puffed.

Gary: I almost hate to think about my worst performance in golf. I remember playing with a group of people I didn't know. I had just walked onto the course one Friday afternoon. These were obviously not very skilled golfers. They were fun-loving and enjoyable people, but they were hackers. I hit my first shot perfectly, long and straight down the middle. They all oohed and aahed and I remember them chattering about wanting me on their team. Soon after that, the wheels came off! I started shanking the ball [a "shank" is sometimes called a lateral shot. Instead of going straight, the ball actually travels almost at a ninety degree angle to the right. It occurs when the ball is hit on the very inside of the heel of the golf club and when the swing is going away from the golfer as opposed to going down the target line]. I couldn't stop shanking the ball. It seemed that no matter what I did, the ball would either shank or half-shank. These guys that I was playing with started giving me advice! Yet, if my game was even semi-normal, I would play far better than any

> of them. I remember them asking for my scores at the end of each hole a few times. I kept telling them that I didn't want to keep track of the score. I had intended on playing eighteen holes that day but I walked off the course after nine holes. It just felt horrible! It was as if I knew nothing about playing golf and would never play a decent game again in my life.

He goes on to say, "A butterfly swimmer captures the blending of self and the experience that occurs with the following comment: 'I couldn't feel any pain, which is really weird, for me...take away the pain and it is effortless...my whole body was doing it with ease.'"

Research by Patrick Cohn confirms the common experience of effortlessness and automaticity during peak performances. Cohn's elite golfers reported that their best performances were automatic and required little or no conscious thought during execution. The golfers reported being unconcerned with mechanical thoughts and feelings typically associated with the early stages of learning a skill. One golfer said, "It was easy; everything felt natural." Another golfer reported, "The swing was just smooth, flowing and just there. I didn't have to work at it all."

Acutely Aware

Athletes sometimes report an acute awareness of their own bodies and/or the actions of other athletes around them during peak experiences (Renee noted this in Exercise 3-1). They feel complete harmony with the sporting environment. Their awareness also remains acutely in the present.

Ravizza quoted a lacrosse player who captured the essence of this type of awareness: "It was a world within a world...focus right there. I was not aware of the external. My concentration was so great I didn't think of anything else."

Charles Garfield and Hal Bennett described this awareness as being "in the cocoon." It's a feeling of being completely detached from the external environment and any distractions. Sometimes athletes report feeling that time slows down during peak experiences. They also feel extremely sensitive to critical elements of the sport. Other athletes report a sense of oneness with their sport, an integration.

Ravizza quoted an Olympic cyclist describing that integration, "I am at one with everything...There is no distinction between myself, the bicycle, track, speed or anything. There is a oneness with everything."

Sometimes baseball players during peak performance perceive the ball as moving in slow motion and seeming larger than it really is. One baseball player once told me, "When I'm really 'on' that ball looks like it's a beach ball floating to the plate." Gymnasts may perceive the balance beam to be wider than it really is. The ability to anticipate the movements of opposing team members seems accentuated. Opponents seem to be moving more slowly; an athlete's visual field seems to encompass everything.

Relaxed

Many athletes describe both mental and physical relaxation as a major part of peak experiences and performances. They talk about a sense of inner calm. Muscles feel loose and movements feel fluid and sure. Consider these quotes from Cohn's elite golfers:

"I was just really relaxed. I had no unnecessary thoughts, totally relaxed like I was in a bubble, no one could get in there…There was no rapid heartbeat or tingling in my hands. There was very little tension compared to what I usually have…I was so relaxed. I just let it happen and it happened…I didn't force any shots. The shoulders weren't tight and I had a good pace walking."

Controlled

Athletes report that their minds and bodies seemed to perform correctly, but they note no sense of imposing control. The control just seems very natural, related both to themselves and their performances. They often report effortless performances, just as they want them to emerge. Athletes also perceive unusual levels of control over emotions, thoughts and arousal levels.

Ravizza quoted a football player's describing his peak experience: "Things were under control; my body could do anything…it was almost like my body was not there. Everything out there could in no way affect me. I could do anything I wanted."

Cohn's golfers often felt a remarkable sense of control during peak performances and experiences:

"I felt I was in control of everything around me. I didn't think about the competition…I knew I was beating them but I didn't let that bother me or get me excited…"

"I felt I was in complete control. I knew exactly what I wanted to do on every shot perfectly…I had a perfect plan for every shot…I was in control of my thoughts. I was thinking about what I wanted to."

"If I made an eagle, I was still going to be in control. I wasn't going to get excited; and if I made a double bogie, I was still going to be in control of my emotions, actions and physical responses to each shot."

Very Positive and Confident, Inspired

During peak experiences, athletes usually report having positive, optimistic attitudes and feeling very confident. They feel capable of maintaining their poise and using their strength effectively even during challenging situations.

Micki King was the only diver from the USA who returned from the 1968 Olympic Games to compete in the 1972 Games. She won an Olympic gold medal in 1972. Her description of the way she dove during those 1972 games shows the power of positive thinking, "I know there is a moment when 'all systems are go.' I can feel it. Standing there, thinking over my dive, I feel my legs tingle. I take a deep breath. All that tingling goes away and a sort of calm comes over me. When that calm reaches me, I am ready to go and *I'm not going to miss.*"

Some of Cohn's elite golfers described their senses of self-confidence during peak experiences:

"Confidence is to know that I can do what I want to do and that I am better than anyone else out there. I have no reason to fear other people."

"Every time I got over the ball, I just swung free and knew where the ball was going before I hit it. I knew it was going at the hole. I would say that 95 percent to 98 percent of the time it was going at the hole…there was no doubt over any shot or putt."

"I didn't think there was any way that I was going to miss a shot. I put fear aside…and my main thoughts were good thoughts. I knew I was going to play well."

"I just knew I could do it…just feel it—it's almost an invincible feeling—you know that it is going your way. I'll tell you what: I almost won the US Open that day."

Fearless

During peak experiences, athletes strive for excellence, undaunted by past mistakes and not worrying about the possibility of failure. Ravizza suggested that when athletes fear failure, they cannot concentrate effectively. Part of their concentration focuses on evaluating on how they're doing and avoiding trouble rather than on their ongoing performance.

Cohn's golfers reported experiencing no fear when playing in the zone:

"I don't think I saw any bunkers or other trouble. I don't remember seeing any bunkers around the greens. I don't remember seeing any trouble around the greens, or fairway traps, or any water."

"I got to a point where I no longer feared a bad shot. I no longer worried about a bad shot or concerned myself with a bad shot. I just knew at that time I was never going to hit another bad shot that round."

"I didn't have a whole lot of fear starting out, but [as the round progressed] I didn't have any fear at all. And so when I say relaxed, I was not worried about anything mentally...I felt I had nothing to lose and I was in really good shape."

Joyful

Peak experiences are described as highly energetic states that include feelings of joy, ecstasy, intensity and fun. According to Ravizza, a downhill skier dramatically captured this aspect of peak experience: "I felt like I was radiating in every direction, not with pressure but with joy. I felt a tremendous amount of heat. I was totally filled up with joy like a helium balloon, and it was fantastic."

Cohn's golfers also reported experiencing a great deal of fun during their peak performances:

"I felt so free. For three hours I had mastered something I had worked for for so long. I was in complete control of everything. It was the most secure, most safe, most exhilarating feeling I have ever had. It was just wonderful."

"I was having fun because I was playing so great and fulfilling my dreams, knowing that you have worked so hard and knowing in your mind that you should have won more tournaments in the past."

"I was having a really good time. I was really enjoying what I was doing...the enjoyment was I was winning the battle with myself...I mean that's fun, and I had that feeling throughout the day."

Peak experiences feel effortless or automatic, maximally aware, relaxed (mentally and physically), well-controlled, confident, optimistic, fearless and extremely positive. Several sports psychologists have created stories that summarize typical peak experiences. Consider the following examples, and try to recall episodes in your own life that seem comparable:

"I was playing possessed, yet in complete control. Time itself seemed to slow down; so [I] never felt rushed. [I] played with profound intensity, total concentration, and an enthusiasm that bordered on joy."

"I felt very relaxed but I was energized and feeling strong. I enjoyed the tennis competition and was not afraid to lose. In fact, I felt a sense of calmness and quiet inside and my strokes just seemed to flow automatically. I really wasn't thinking about my shots and what I needed to do; it just seemed to happen naturally. My shots did not feel rushed; in fact, the ball seemed to slow down and I felt as if I could do almost anything. I was totally into the match, yet I was not consciously trying to concentrate. I was aware of everything but distracted by nothing. I knew my shots were going in and I felt confident and in control."

Weight controllers can get to this level of ease with the process of losing weight and, perhaps more so, with the process of maintaining weight loss. Researchers who study very successful weight controllers, particularly James Hill and Rena Wing, co-founders of The National Weight Control Registry, began asking highly successful weight controllers lots of questions in 1994. They and their colleagues published dozens of papers on these successful people to help point the way to success for others. In one study, they asked these masters of weight control (their average weight loss was sixty pounds, maintained for an average of five years) if they found the process easier over time. Sure enough, the masters rated the process significantly easier at year six than year three, and year three significantly easier than the first year of success. A study by my colleagues and I showed that one of the final stages associated with success, "Acceptance," includes a profound acceptance and a peaceful sense of resolve. Putting these insights about weight control together, you can recognize parts of peak experience and peak performance. As weight controllers master the process over a period of years, they find it easier and feel more peaceful and accepting about the

---

Weight Controller–Athlete Parallel #2:
PEAK PERFORMANCE

- Peak performances for athletes feel easy, relaxed, confident, aware, well-controlled, fearless and extremely positive.
- Masterful weight controllers find the process easier over time and feel more peaceful and accepting of the challenges than when they had less experience.

challenges involved. Peak performances and experiences have parallel characteristics: ease, joy and confidence.

Obviously, athletes love peak experiences. Legendary golfer Ben Hogan reported hitting only a few perfect shots in his lifetime! Hogan's report does *not* coincide with his actual performances. He won eight major golf championships and dozens of others. That should have produced more than a couple of peak experiences, but Hogan did not feel it that way. For most athletes, however, peak experiences accompany great performances. This makes peak experience a very desirable goal. When athletes take deliberate steps to achieve peak experiences, their performances can improve dramatically.

What steps can you take to achieve more peak experiences? The first step involves a certain attitude or orientation toward goal-setting.

GOAL ORIENTATION FOR PEAK PERFORMANCE

Mastery-oriented goal setting means you tend to focus on the process, not just the outcome of the competition, when performing in a game or sport. You can either set process goals or outcome goals in sports, games and weight control. In the current analysis, goal setting is viewed as a personal style. Some people tend to use mastery or process type goals; others prefer outcome or competitive goals. Which goal orientation do you think produces the best outcomes?

Sports psychologist Joan Duda's research indicates that mastery-oriented athletes practiced their sports more in their spare time than did competitive-oriented athletes. Damon Burton found that swimmers who were taught to use a mastery orientation expended more effort than swimmers without training in mastery orientation who set mainly competitive goals. This makes sense. If you focus on mastery, you focus on improving and building your skills. This encourages you to work hard to bring your skills to higher levels. If you focus on beating your opponents (competitive orientation), you will be satisfied by winning more than by improving skills. What happens when you play weak opponents? Competitively-oriented athletes may only push hard enough to win. Their skills could stagnate. They also may feel especially distraught when they lose. Mastery-oriented folks would feel great if they won, but also if they met their process or mastery goals.

Complete Exercise 3-2 now to help you analyze your own goal orientation.

> ### Exercise 3-2: Mastery vs. Competitive Goal Orientations
>
> *Think about your best performances in any sport or game. Then complete the following questions about that performance, rating the degree to which you focused on each of the points listed (items 1-10). Rate the item as a 10 if you focused a great deal on that item or if the statement characterizes your performance extremely well; rate a 1 if that item does not indicate a focus or your attention or describe your reaction to your performance well at all.*
>
> **Rating**
> When I performed my best I:
> 1) learned a new skill _____
> 2) worked really hard _____
> 3) did my very best _____
> 4) learned something fun _____
> 5) focused on personal improvement much more than winning _____
>
> 1-5 Total _____
>
> 6) realized I was the best _____
> 7) noticed that others were messing up _____
> 8) focused on outperforming my opponents _____
> 9) realized that winning was very important to me _____
> 10) realized I had more skills than others _____
>
> 6-10 Total _____

To score: Add the numbers corresponding to the ratings for questions 1 through 5. This total provides your *mastery goal orientation* score. Adding ratings for 6 through 10 provides your score for *competitiveness goal orientation*. Higher numbers indicate stronger feelings toward each goal orientation. Is your mastery orientation higher than your competitiveness goal orientation? Or vice versa?

The recommendation from these studies is clear: *Focus on mastery or process goals in order to perform your best.* In addition, other studies show that using both outcome and process goals together maximizes performance. Unfortunately, this is much easier said than done. Our culture wants athletes to "go for the gold." We are an outcome-oriented society,

> **Weight Controller–Athlete Parallel #3:**
> *PROCESS AND OUTCOME GOALS*
> - Athletes perform best when they use both process (mastery-oriented) and outcome (competition-oriented) goals.
> - Weight controllers benefit from using both process and outcome goals.

but you can still strive to win with a mastery orientation. Focus on the skills and efforts required to make yourself a winner, not just on winning.

Let's draw some parallels to weight control. You could focus on the number on the scale alone. Whatever it takes to get that number where you want it becomes secondary to getting that number to move in the right direction. Unfortunately, weight fluctuates due to many things, including the amount of salt you eat, the amount of sweating you've done and even the time of day. If you get on a scale with an outcome orientation, you can get very upset when the number doesn't cooperate. That would happen regardless of the reason for the fluctuation in your weight. That upset reaction has led some people to give up trying altogether.

You could also focus on the amount of fat you're consuming, the amount of steps you accumulate on a pedometer and other elements of the process of losing weight. Then, if the scale shows you something other than weight loss, you can see if your process met your standards. If you did exercise adequately and ate very little fat, then you can realize that the number on the scale will probably decrease in a day or two. If the process meets your standard as a weight controller, it protects you from the normal fluctuations in outcomes. So, just like in sports or games, using both process and outcome goals can improve your effectiveness in weight control. Research supports this assertion by demonstrating the importance of both daily self-monitoring (recording of food, for example) and daily self-weighing.

TALENT VS. PRACTICE

Three other keys to peak performance are: practice, practice and practice! Practice deserves this emphasis when you consider methods of maximizing your sport performance. Yet, many people argue that no amount or type of practice can produce outstanding performance if you don't have the talent. The notion that inherited talent is much more important than practice deserves a closer look.

Influential writers have sung the praises of inherited talent for centuries. For example, in Edward Young's famous article on the origin of creativity, "Conjectures on Original Composition," he argued that, "An *Original* may be said to be of vegetable nature: It rises spontaneously from the vital root of Genius; it *grows,* it is not *made.*"

Young's view was that genius and talent were born. Talent was considered independent of learning and training. This makes talent opposite to acquired skill. Anders Ericsson and Neil Charness noted that similar ideas were first espoused by painter Georgio Vasari in 1568. In his classic book, *The Lives of the Artists,* Vasari attempted to provide biographies of famous artists. Vasari's *Lives* fostered the idea that artists, like himself, were granted special gifts by God and, therefore, should be entitled to recognition, payment and abiding respect.

Vasari tried to identify early signs of talent and ability in the artists he described. When facts were missing, Vasari simply added or distorted material. For example, Vasari claimed that his own first public showing of his unusual talents occurred when he was nine. Historians now know that he was thirteen at that event. Vasari also invented linkages between outstanding artists of his day and earlier great artists. He emphasized that talent came from God, not practice. For example, Vasari described Michelangelo's famous painting, the *Final Judgment,* as "the great example sent by God to men so that they can perceive what can be done when intellects of the highest grade descend upon the earth."

Most people today still believe this ancient view of talent. For example, one Howard Gardner, an influential scientist, wrote, "it seems possible that [extraordinary talent in children] is primarily hereditary, and…needs as little external stimulation as does walking and talking in the normal child."

What percentage would you assign to inherited talent versus trained skill? In other words, what percentage of current skill levels in your favorite athletes came from their genetic tendencies versus learned skills via instruction and practice? If you believe that most athletic skills emerge from inherited talent, carefully consider the following points, derived from some fascinating articles written by K. Anders Ericsson and his colleagues. More recent research underscores the principles Ericsson and associates described in the 1990s (Bruce, Farrow and Raynor, 2013). Here are some startling facts:

Implications for Weight Controller-Athletes

- Most child prodigies do *not* become exceptional performers as adults. If talent dominated as the cause of adult athletic performance, you would expect most prodigies to excel as adults.
- The vast majority of exceptional adult performers were never child prodigies. Many musicians show an early interest in music. They rarely show exceptional skill or talent. But, they almost always start instruction early and increase their performance due to sustaining a high level of training throughout their lives.
- László and Klara Polgár used their own children to demonstrate the ability of instruction and practice, not talent per se, to determine exceptional performance. As part of an educational experiment, László and Klara Polgár raised one of their daughters to become the youngest international chess Grand Master ever. She was even younger than Bobby Fischer, the famous American chess whiz who was the youngest male who achieved that exceptional level of performance. In 1992, the three Polgár daughters were ranked first, second and sixth in the world among female chess players.
- *Savants* are individuals with low levels of general intellectual functioning but who can perform at very high levels in certain special tasks. Many people use the existence of these savants as evidence for the argument that exceptional skills come from exceptional inborn abilities. Careful study of these special talents shows that opportunities, support and strong encouragement for learning often preceded the development of savants' skills by years or even decades. For example, savants who can name the day of the week of an arbitrary date (for example, October 2, 1950) generate their answers using methods that can be reproduced by college students after a few weeks of training. Even music savants, who supposedly can play a piece of music perfectly after a single hearing, show dramatic limitations in these abilities. These limitations are inconsistent with an over-emphasis on inborn talent. Music savants cannot readily imitate unfamiliar sequences of music that violate typical Western scale structures.
- Highly skilled chess players can reproduce locations of all the chess pieces almost perfectly after observing a chess game for a few seconds. Weaker chess players cannot do this. However, research by Chase and Simon showed that this special "talent" to memorize disappeared when chess positions were created

with randomly arranged pieces. Superior memory depends very definitely on perceiving meaningful patterns and relations. Highly skilled chess players have far more experience with a wide variety of positions. These well-developed skills promote better memory of meaningful patterns of chess pieces.

- The average IQ of Grand Masters in chess is about that of an average college student. Grand Masters also do not differ in IQ from average club chess players. These findings would surprise those who argue that talent determines performance.
- The human body is remarkably adaptable. The number of capillaries supplying blood to muscle fibers changes after a few weeks of training. Muscle fibers can change from fast twitch to slow twitch and vice versa, depending on practice levels. Fast twitch muscles facilitate bursts of speed while slow twitch muscles maximize endurance. Changes in lung capacity, bone density, heart size and aerobic capacity increase when training increases. Researchers have even found that differences in the percentages of slow twitch fibers in athletes' muscles occur only for muscles specifically trained for their sports. For example, the legs in runners and back muscles of kayakers show these changes. Untrained muscles do not show these changes.
- Experts and non-experts do not differ on measures of general skills that seem clearly related to expert performance of a specific skill. For example, a recent study of expert versus non-expert pianists (of similar age) showed that the experts and the lesser players performed similarly on two different tasks that measured reaction times and speed of hand movements. Those who advocate for the vital role of talent would have expected differences in these related tasks between experts and non-experts. The findings suggest that experts developed very domain-specific skills via practice.
- Comparisons of experts versus non-experts in varying domains—tennis players, field-hockey players, typists, medical diagnosticians and chess players—reveal something very interesting and consistent across all of them. Experts do not differ from non-experts in general cognitive or memory skills. The differences between these groups of experts versus non-experts were restricted to their domains of expertise. Experts can anticipate future movements or actions only in their

domains much better than non-experts. For example, expert tennis players can use such early cues as the location of an opponent's arms and racket to predict accurately where a tennis ball will hit in the service area. Elite field-hockey players can predict where the ball will go by looking at pictures of attacking field hockey players. These pictures showed the position of the hockey players even before their sticks made contact with the ball.

- Elite performers consistently differ from their non-elite peers in the amount and intensity of their deliberate practice. For example, runners at the national level have been found to train 4.9 times per week; runners at regional and local levels trained 4.2 and 3.2 times per week, respectively. Outcomes of marathon races can be predicted with a great deal of accuracy from the regularity and amount of practice during the nine weeks prior to the race. Practice seems to predict performance, suggesting the paramount role of learning and experience over talent.

Convinced? The evidence is both remarkable and overwhelming. Maximum athletic performance comes from maximum deliberate practice. No amount of inborn genetic ability can overcome inadequate practice. Most people think that chess masters are particularly good examples of geniuses. It's simply hard to fathom how people could play such an intricate game with tremendous speed and precision if they weren't blessed with extraordinary intellectual gifts.

Among chess masters, Bobby Fischer and Judit Polgár are classic examples of those considered geniuses. These two individuals attained their international Grand Master status at fifteen, the youngest recorded age in history. Bobby Fischer learned the rules of chess at age six. During that same year, he began studying his first book of chess games. At age seven, Fischer got in touch with the president of the Brooklyn Chess Club, who tutored him every week for several years. At age twelve, Fischer joined one of the best chess clubs in the world, the Manhattan Chess Club. Around that time he started close interactions with chess master Jack Collins. He met with Collins several times a week and got free access to Collins's outstanding library of chess books. Fischer began collecting his own chess books and, in 1973 (at the time of his international acclaim), he had about four hundred books and thousands of magazines and journals all about chess. According to some very knowledgeable chess experts, Bobby Fischer became the best-educated chess theoretician in modern times.

Judit Polgár's father introduced her to chess and tutored her from the time she was four or five. Judit did not attend regular school and was allowed to spend all of her time with her parents, who were both teachers and chess experts.

Are Bobby Fischer and Judit Polgár talented geniuses or examples of what a combination of commitment plus nurturance plus practice can really do? Like Fischer and Polgár, expert performers in a wide variety of domains spend about twenty-five hours per week in deliberate practice and about fifty to sixty hours per week on domain-related activities. For example, elite distance runners often run twice a day and cover distances from forty-five to two hundred miles per week every week of the year. Their normal days of practice consist of a session in the morning and a more strenuous session in the afternoon, including many hours for preparation, warm-up, massage and other related activities. Similar estimates are reported for swimming and cycling.

Implications for Weight Controllers

Practice seems far more powerful as a determinant of skilled athletic performance than the much more elusive quality of talent. It seems that under the right conditions, almost anyone could become an excellent athlete, chess player or pianist. Weight controllers might sometimes believe that they do not have the requisite personality or skills to master the challenges of losing weight. Those doubts resemble the frustrations that all athletes feel when they struggle to perform. These findings about the power of practice argue that it takes a willingness to put in the time to master your chosen domain to succeed. If you're willing to work at it, and you know what to do, you can become a masterful weight controller.

Weight Controller–Athlete Parallel #4:
PRACTICE DETERMINES OUTCOME MORE THAN TALENT
- Talent determines performance far less than most people think.
- Lots of practice and good instruction lead to great performances.
- If weight controllers have the willingness to work hard to overcome inevitable frustrations, they can succeed. They do not require a particular personality or talent to master the process.

UNDERSTANDING PRACTICE

What makes practice so critical? How do people use practice to learn? How is practice for novices different from practice for experts? The answers to these questions emerge once you understand the phases of learning that lead to expert performance.

To identify phases of learning, try to recall exactly how you learned to play your favorite sport or musical instrument. Review all of the circumstances surrounding your first attempts. Recall the kind of encouragement you received from friends and family. What sort of instruction did you receive, if any? How often did you play or practice? Can you identify phases or stages in your learning or skill development? Here is a story told to me by one of my clients. See if you can identify some similar phases of your own learning.

"I can't remember when I first picked up a tennis racket. Maybe I was four or five years old. My older brother loved to play tennis. I remember how much fun it was to just hit the ball with the racket and watch it go what seemed like a mile in the air. I used to play with that thing in the schoolyard while my brother was doing something else. My brother was several years older than I, so he didn't let me play against him for quite a while. But I would accompany him to the tennis court.

"Eventually, my parents gave me my own tennis racket. The first one was a hand-me-down from my brother. One of the strings was broken, but I didn't seem to mind. I remember starting to play primitive tennis games with my friends when I was about six or seven years old. Our older brothers and sisters would have fairly intense games (at least it looked that way to us) on nearby courts. We would hack it around on our own court and get yelled at by our siblings for knocking too many balls in their courts. I had two or three friends who liked to do this kind of thing with me. We would also sometimes take our rackets and make up a game by hitting the ball against a schoolyard wall or handball court. (I grew up in a big city and walls were more available to us than tennis courts). We seemed to gain more and more control over the ball in just a few months of doing these things.

"I remember starting to read about tennis just about as soon as I could read. I would read my brother's tennis magazines and information about tennis players in the newspapers. Every spring I started to look forward to the tennis season beginning (we had no indoor courts available to us) with increased enthusiasm. My brother saw that I was very interested and began teaching me what he knew. When I was about eight or nine, he started letting me play against him. He would take it easy on me and we started to have fun competing. Some of my friends also competed with me. At this point I still hadn't received any formal tennis lessons. I always regret that and think that it could have helped me a lot at that point.

"I eventually made it to my high school tennis team where I finally got some useful direction. It was a little difficult to do some of the things suggested to me by my coach (especially modifications in grip). My tennis game seemed to get worse before it got better whenever I made some of the changes he suggested. Nevertheless, I seemed to get better and better throughout high school. I made more and more of a commitment to tennis and was practicing virtually every day by the time I reached college. I played for my college team and tennis became a huge part of my life."

THREE PHASES OF LEARNING

Phase 1: Playful Initiation

This story illustrates the attitude of playfulness in the early phases of learning. Figure 3-1 shows Bernard Bloom's analysis of the three phases that experts experience when developing their skills. The first phase begins with the individual's introduction to his or her sport or activity and ends with formal instruction and deliberate practice. This early phase involves playful activities in the sport. The child picks up the tennis racket and smacks the ball in the air. He or she does this over and over again. Parents or siblings see this happening and provide encouragement. The fast runner is recognized and entered into early competitions for fun. The enthusiastic golfer is brought to a driving range to

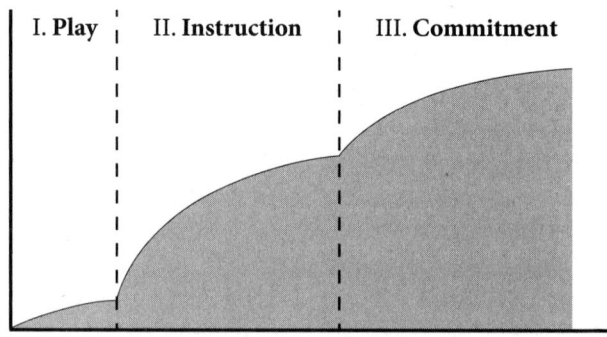

Figure 3-1. Bloom's (1985) three phases of development toward adult expertise.

accompany a parent. Ben Crenshaw, the two-time Masters champion and now world-class golf course architect, received his first lesson from a legendary teaching pro, Harvey Penick. Mr. Penick told the seven year-old Ben, "Here you go. Take this ball and this chipping club and putter and go to that practice green over there. Chip the ball onto the green and putt it into the hole. Come back to me when you are pretty good at doing that. Have fun with it."

Phase 2: Instruction Begins

Bloom's second phase begins with more systematic instruction and deliberate practice. Children become involved in team sports. They receive coaching from people who are knowledgeable in the sport. They begin to play and practice more systematically. They start reading and thinking about the sport on a more regular basis. This instructional phase ends when the athlete becomes committed to full-time involvement with the sport. Most readers of this book have not experienced the next phase, full-time commitment. Avid athletes, unlike experts, participate very seriously, but without taking twenty-five or more hours per week to get to the next level. You may, however, find it useful to learn about this next phase. Just imagine where your skills could have gone if you put in that amount of time and focus.

Phase 3: Full-time Commitment

Expert performers design their lives to optimize their practice schedules. In most domains, including sports performance, experts seem to practice very deliberately for approximately *four hours a day*. This includes practicing every day—including weekends and holidays. Elite performers usually practice most frequently during the morning, when they have the greatest capacity for complex, demanding activity. Practice when athletes are fatigued and unfocused is not only wasteful but possibly harmful.

As you can see, the change from the instruction phase to the full-time commitment phase is huge. That is probably why most avid athletes never experience this phase. Full-time involvement requires tremendous dedication to the sport. The level of competition greatly increases, the intensity heightens, the demands on the body multiply and the demands on the family also grow. There are also considerable risks involved. Athletes in this phase essentially put all of their eggs in one basket. It's a gamble on their abilities to accomplish high-level goals. They sacrifice other paths they could have taken and other skills that they could have developed. This is a very serious phase. It can take some of the fun out of the sport. Certainly, some of the previously quoted writers noticed changes from their early playful, joyful days to the more intense and rigorous days of this final commitment.

Implications for Weight Controllers

It may well take something similar to Phase 3, intensive commitment, to succeed as a weight controller. That's probably closer to the involvement necessary to succeed than the instructional level in Phase 2.

COGNITIVE, ASSOCIATIVE OR AUTONOMOUS PROCESSES IN LEARNING

Bloom's three phases of learning show how some athletes go from just playing and enjoying a sport to mastering it. Within those phases, athletes change the connection between their thoughts and actions. Let's consider that evolution as another way of understanding the development of mastery.

Cognitive Processing

Cognitive processing of information dominates Bloom's first playful phase and usually the instructional phase, as well. Athletes use vision as their primary tool during this time. They visualize the movements of their arms and legs after watching others. Instructors must tell athletes specifically what to look for so they can incorporate the knowledge they see into something they can reproduce.

Associative Learning

The associative or intermediate step in learning skills takes much longer than the cognitive phase. It ranges from perhaps a few hours to learn simple skills to many years for mastering complex ones. Fischman and Oxendine suggested that during this phase the learner practices the skill to the point that it is performed accurately and consistently. Instruction focuses more on encouraging practice and providing constructive feedback. During this phase athletes learn more by feel than by vision. After many, many practice trials, athletes come to associate the feel of their movements with the outcomes that these movements produce. This association of feel with results is what gives the associative phase its name.

During associative learning, athletes gradually decrease extra movements and errors. They tend to improve their speed, accuracy, coordination and consistency. By the end of the associative phase, athletes begin to develop mastery.

Autonomous or Advanced

In the final step to learning a skill, the autonomous or advanced phase, athletes can perform skills with high levels of proficiency and mastery. Performance has become quite automatic and feel-oriented. For example, what would happen to your sport performance if you focused very deliberately on how you executed each element in it? If you are an avid tennis player, consider focusing on each element of the service: the toss of the ball, shoulder position, racket back, grip pressure, etc. Thinking of these components while attempting to serve would interfere with the smoothness and power of the serve. Getting very mechanically focused at any high-speed movement often worsens outcomes.

LeBron James provides another example of the automaticity of highly skilled performance. He can dribble the basketball downcourt at full speed, change course by dribbling behind his back without looking at the ball and, simultaneously, plan the best strategy for getting the ball to the hoop. During such a play, he considers the position and movements of his opponents and teammates. He decides whether to deliver a bounce pass to the right or left or fake in one direction or drive to the basket himself. James does this all while dribbling at full speed, giving virtually no thought to the mechanics of dribbling itself. His dribbling has become automatic.

To progress from the cognitive through the associative and arrive at the autonomous phase of learning requires tremendous amounts of practice and usually long periods of time. The amount of time and practice depends somewhat on the ability of the individual, the nature and complexities of the tasks and the learner's efficiency and experiences. Researchers focused on expert performance believe that it requires eight to fifteen years, ten thousand hours and more than a million repetitions to produce high-level performance in major sports such as football, basketball, baseball and gymnastics.

You could raise many questions about the nature of effective deliberate practice. For example, does practice work best when it is very intensive or "massed" as opposed to distributed over time? Other basic questions about practice include, should whole routines or aspects of performance be practiced, or should the parts of the routines that require the most work be the primary focus? Let's consider the answers that science suggests about these questions for athletes and then draw parallels to weight controllers.

MASSED VS. DISTRIBUTED PRACTICE

In 1916 Arthur Murphy taught right-handed subjects how to throw a javelin at a target with their left hands. Each subject made five throws on each of thirty-four days of practice. The massed group practiced five days per week, while the distributed group practiced three times per week. They all practiced the same total number of throws. The group that distributed its practice outperformed the massed practice group. Subjects who practiced three times a week were more accurate hitting the target after thirty-four days of practice than the massed practice group. The distributed practice group was still better than the massed practice group even during a re-testing three months later.

Many studies have examined these effects since Murphy's research was published nearly one hundred years ago. Usually, the outcomes favor distributed instead of massed practice. Why should distributed practice produce better outcomes? Think about the processes of learning discussed in the preceding section for a hint.

Cognitive aspects of learning a task take a certain amount of time. When practice is distributed over days or weeks, learners can use the information that they get through practice more effectively. If practice occurs at a very intense and frequent pace, learners may become confused more easily. They may have difficulty sorting out the information and feedback that they receive in practice.

These findings argue for taking lessons every few days or once a week in the early phases of learning rather than going to a camp or school that provides intensive training on an hourly or daily basis. This is especially important for beginning or intermediate learners. Very experienced avid athletes, however, could incorporate more massed or intensive levels of training and practicing. On the other hand, even experienced athletes might sometimes find themselves overstimulated by information when learning a new technique or aspect of their sports. Under those conditions, they could take more time between instructional sessions.

WHOLE VS. PART PRACTICE

Consider the complexity of most sports skills. For example, think about a gymnast completing a floor exercise. What about a basketball player executing a reverse lay-up or a diver performing a forward double somersault with two twists? How about a novice golfer's thirty-yard pitch shot? Would these athletes benefit most from learning components of these complex skills in small units or should they attempt to execute entire skills and practice "whole learning?"

The decision to practice a skill as a whole or in parts should be based on the nature of the skill and the nature of the learner. In general, the whole learning method produces better outcomes under four conditions:

1. If the skill can be understood in a meaningful way by the learner, whole learning works well.
2. If the skill is relatively safe to practice, then it can be practiced as a whole unit. Consider the relative safety and likelihood of achieving success for certain gymnastics tricks, diving routines, wrestling maneuvers and pole vaulting attempts. The potential for injury and failure make some of these procedures better taught in parts rather than as a whole.
3. When the athlete is highly capable, highly motivated and has an extensive background in the sport, the whole method may produce better outcomes than the part method.
4. The athlete's attention span must be long enough to work with the whole unit rather than a simpler part approach.

These four principles also imply that, *under some conditions*, part practice produces better outcomes. For example, when one particular component causes great difficulty, better results will come from concentrating on that component. This provides additional practice where it is most needed. However, practicing in parts can cause mechanical disruptions in the overall routine. The coach must help the athlete integrate troublesome parts back into the whole skill as smoothly as possible.

Another aspect of whole versus part learning pertains to the *variability* of practicing. For example, should a tennis player use a machine that delivers a tennis ball at exactly the same speed and to the exact same spot to practice forehand and backhand returns of serve? Or, would the tennis player improve faster having a coach serve balls to provide greater variability? Should swimmers practice one type of stroke during practice session A followed by another in practice session B? Or, should the swimmer practice the crawl and butterfly in both sessions?

The answer favors increasing variability for better outcomes. More variable practice conditions imitate actual game conditions better than blocked or more constant practice conditions. In actual game or tournament situations, variability occurs. Practicing under variable conditions, therefore, better prepares the athlete to cope with game or tournament situations. Athletes learn how to switch from one type of stroke to another or to master the changing nature of actual game situations more effectively. They develop greater overall confidence in their abilities to cope with changing circumstances.

All of this suggests that athletes would be better off practicing a variety of components of their sports in each session rather than focusing exclusively on one element. Another advantage to this approach pertains to confidence. The golfer who struggles with lag putts, for example, may gain confidence from practicing chip shots as well as lag putting.

Making Practice Perfect Practice:
A Recap

Ask any real estate agent about the three keys to buying property and you'll often hear: "location, location, location!" The three keys to producing the best athletic performances are: "practice, practice, practice!" Further refinement emphasizes making practice perfect practice. Lots of perfect practice is an absolute must for high levels of performance.

Our culture emphasizes talent but the scientific literature emphasizes the development of skills in practice. If athletes stay with science, they will improve their sports performances more consistently. Science also directs us toward practicing in a distributed way, focusing on whole practice under some conditions and maximizing variability in practice routines. Science also argues for the benefit of guidance and instruction at the highest level available. This may mean shopping around for coaches and instructors who provide useful and positive feedback.

Implications for Weight Controllers

Weight controllers must develop healthy obsessions to succeed. This requires consistent planning, goal setting and execution of certain types of eating, movement and self-monitoring. Athletes require tremendous amounts of certain types of practice. For weight controllers, we can expect experience (practice) with planning and goal setting to produce more effective execution over time. That experience, or practice, can include analyzing the high-risk nature of certain situations (like travel, dining out and parties). It also includes practice or experience with effective coping strategies (like bringing one's own food, reviewing menus online before dining out and requesting certain accommodations from hosts of parties). Practice with eating a very low-fat, low-energy-density diet would also eventually lead to that autonomous, highly committed style of integration, closely akin to a healthy obsession. So, too, would repeated experience with daily movement at a high level lead to a more autonomous healthy obsession over time.

Based on the research pertaining to types of practice, I believe that many weight controllers could benefit from intensive experiences, such as those available in immersion programs (therapeutic camps and residential programs). Weight controllers grapple with their challenges every day for many years. With that degree of experience, they parallel advanced athletes who benefit most from intensive training experiences. Also, immersion programs can replicate the benefits of whole versus part practice. In immersion environments, weight controllers get to live with programs that stress high levels of activity, consistent self-monitoring and very low-fat, calorie-controlled eating. That integrative, holistic approach may prove more useful than working with a trainer on the physical aspects or with a dietitian on the food component.

Within both immersion programs and other support efforts (e.g., self-help groups and cognitive-behavioral therapy groups), it might prove useful to review and role play responses to a wide array of high-risk situations. That suggestion comes from the findings that encourage variability in practice to maximize results.

> **Weight Controller–Athlete Parallel #5:**
> *PERFECT PRACTICE MAKES PERFECT*
>
> 1. Amount of practice determines skilled performance in sports far more than talent.
> 2. Best practices: distributed, whole and variable; but more experienced athletes can do very well with massed and part practices.
> 3. Weight controllers probably do not have to have certain personality types or styles to benefit from experience with planning, problem solving and eating/moving effectively to lose weight.
> 4. Many weight controllers have substantial experience and may, therefore, do well with immersion (massed) treatments and with focusing on improving all aspects of the weight control process at once (whole practice).

CHAPTER 4

Becoming Overweight— Causes and Fixes

This chapter addresses the question:
"Since I'm not a food addict, what caused my weight problem?"

We will consider the primary causes of weight problems and how best to correct them. You know at this point that as a weight controller-athlete you can overcome biological and other challenges. Success does not require special talents, just as the concept of talent fails to predict athletic accomplishment as well as skill and hard work do. However, we benefit from knowledge of challenges, similarly to how athletes benefit from knowing the details about how to master their sports. All elite athletes understand the requirements of their training regimens and equipment. Masterful weight controllers benefit by learning the causes of weight gain and the best approaches to lose weight.

Before focusing specifically on weight control, let's discuss some psychological principles or factors that predict and control behavior more generally. These will help you create a foundation of knowledge to help frame the presentation about weight loss. Every sport has fundamentals. For example, a famous instructor and friend of mine, Dr. DeDe Owens, described the fundamentals of the golf swing as: grip, posture and pivot (or how a golfer turns away from the ball to generate power). When golfers struggle with their swings, they go back to those fundamentals to figure out the cause of the swing fault and the fix for it. Psychology provides the fundamental knowledge required to understand how and why people gain and lose weight in much the same way.

PSYCHOLOGY: FACTORS THAT IMPACT BEHAVIOR, INCLUDING BEHAVIOR CHANGE

Three Response Systems

Consider any complex behavior or emotion, like anxiety. What occurs to you when you think about the last time you felt anxious? Maybe you had to give a talk to colleagues. Maybe you had to make a five-foot putt to win a hole or confront a boss or loved one about a problem. Try describing that anxiety. You could describe it in terms of behaviors, like saying "Uh" frequently or moving around in a jittery way. You could also describe the feeling itself. Anxiety feels unpleasant, queasy or uneasy. You could also describe thoughts, like doubting yourself, worrying or expecting problems and more unpleasantness. Finally, anxiety often has a biological response or two like excess sweating, rapid breathing or your heart pounding.

Psychologist Peter Lang did a series of landmark studies showing that the three response systems pictured in Figure 4-1 function in a related way during emotional reactions, but also quite independently of one another at times. Someone giving a speech for example, may look calm to the audience but afterwards report tremendously unpleasant feelings and thoughts. The calm behavior in this case occurred independently from the thoughts and feelings. This applies directly to weight control. Some weight controllers may eat problematic foods, in quantities beyond their goals, and report feeling unconcerned about that deviation from the plan. Others could react with tremendous negative emotion when drifting away from plans and goals. It helps

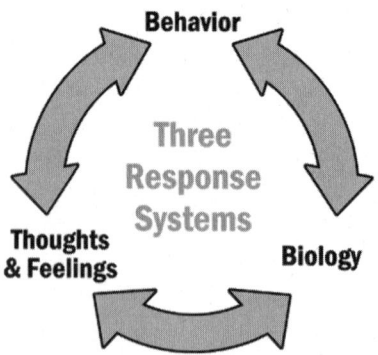

Figure 4-1. Three response systems function somewhat independently.

to know, when thinking about approaches to losing weight, that some or all three response systems can impact the outcome of the effort. In the next chapters, we'll discuss how the Wellspring Plan places greater emphasis on behaviors and biology and less emphasis on certain types of thoughts and feelings than other approaches. The food addict perspective clearly emphasizes the feelings side of this response wheel (emotional distress causes over-eating) and de-emphasizes the other parts of the three response systems.

Biological, Social-Environmental and Intra-personal Determinants of Behavior

Figure 4-2 shows that these three factors influence our behaviors in powerful ways. Biology affects us every day. For example, our genetics can greatly impact our height, skin color, personality and tendency to gain weight easily. The culture in which we live affects us, too. Some of us have enough money and accessibility to stores and restaurants so that we can buy high-quality, very low-fat foods or also high-fat, problematic foods. Clearly family and friends impact us, too. If we have very active athletic families and friends, getting and staying active becomes a natural and ingrained part of our lifestyles. Sedentary friends and family can affect us in the opposite direction. Finally, we also have active inner (or intra-personal) lives. Figure 4-2 summarizes these three major influences on behavior.

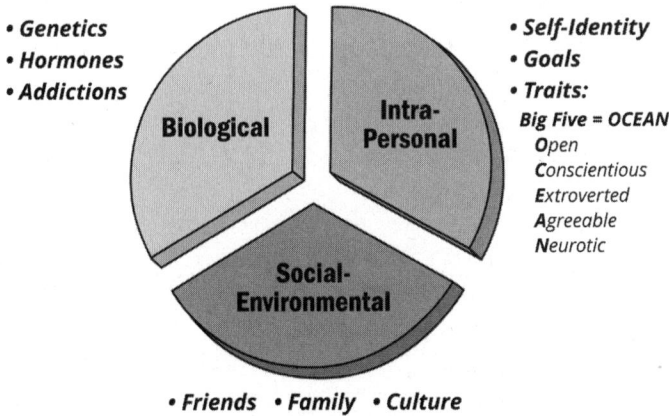

Figure 4-2. Three major influences on behavior: biological, social-environmental and intra-personal.

The food addict approach overemphasizes our intra-personal lives. It essentially argues that emotional problems cause overweight people to binge eat to cope with the stresses and strains of life. That ignores the biological realities of obesity, such as genetic factors and cultural influences, like the over-abundance of cheap, heavily-advertised, high-fat foods on every street corner.

Our identities and goals also impact us. Think of the most athletic people you know. When such people describe themselves, they usually start talking about their sports with big smiles on their faces. Weight controllers can either set goals to change or not. For example, research shows that when people wear pedometers to measure their steps, those who also set goals (like 10,000 steps per day) record significantly more steps on average than those who do not set specific goals.

Personality traits are relatively enduring characteristics that affect our behaviors and attitudes in certain ways in many situations. Paul Costa and Robert McCrae at the National Institutes of Health, Warren Norman at the University of Michigan and Lewis Goldberg at the University of Oregon discovered that five broad dimensions of personality, called the Big Five, seem to work well to describe our general tendencies to behave in predictable ways. The researchers figured this out by asking thousands of people hundreds of questions and then analyzing the data with a statistical procedure that grouped the responses into their simplest form (using factor analysis). The Big Five has become the most widely accepted and used model of personality by researchers.

The acronym OCEAN summarizes the names of the Big Five: openness to experiences, conscientiousness, extraversion, agreeableness and neuroticism (emotional instability vs. stability). Complete Exercise 4-1 to see the defining terms for each of the Big Five and also to get an estimate of your Big Five tendencies.

Several remarkable studies have shown that one of these traits predicts weight status decades after people have completed such personality tests as the one in Exercise 4-1. Which do you think predicts relatively lower weights over time? If you guessed conscientiousness, then you got it right. In 2013, Sarah Hamson and her colleagues reported a forty-year follow-up study conducted in Hawaii. Seven hundred and fifty-three ten-year-old children had their Big Five traits assessed by teachers; then, forty years later, health professionals measured a variety of things. Those people whom the teachers rated low in

> **Exercise 4-1: Big Five Personality Test**
>
> Answer the next ten questions, based on a brief version of a questionnaire about the Big Five personality traits by Samuel Gosling and colleagues at the University of Texas. Use this rating scale to answer the questions:
>
>   1= Disagree Strongly
>   2 = Disagree
>   3 = Disagree Somewhat
>   4 = Neither Agree nor Disagree
>   5 = Agree Somewhat
>   6 = Agree
>   7 = Agree Strongly
>
> I see myself as:
>   1. Extraverted, socially dominant, full of enthusiasm   _____
>   2. Not shy or reserved   _____
>   3. Not overly critical and argumentative   _____
>   4. Sympathetic and warm   _____
>   5. Open to new experiences   _____
>   6. Unconventional and creative   _____
>   7. Well organized, careful and responsible   _____
>   8. Dependable and self-disciplined   _____
>   9. Emotionally unstable   _____
>   10. Easily upset, sometimes anxious or depressed   _____
>
> High scores on the following items suggest tendencies toward the trait listed before them: Extraverted:1, 2; agreeable: 3,4; open: 5,6; conscientious: 7,8; neurotic: 9,10.

conscientiousness as ten-year-olds tended later in life to have higher blood pressure, higher cholesterol and higher Body Mass Indexes (a standard measure of weight divided by height). People who generally tended to persevere in the face of challenges, complete tasks in disciplined and well-organized ways, seemed to manage their health better than people who scored high on other traits.

CAUSES OF OBESITY

Understanding the three response systems (behavior, thoughts and feelings, biology) and the three primary influences on behavior (social-environmental, biological and intra-personal) sets the stage for delving into the causes of excess weight gain. Let's consider the possible causes of weight problems from that perspective, including an analysis of the social-environmental factors and the other influences we just reviewed.

THE "OBESOGENIC" ENVIRONMENT

About ten years ago, experts began referring to our culture as "obesogenic." This means that it has become the natural response to our social environment, and the culture of most developed countries, to gain excess amounts of weight over time. Our social environment essentially nurtures obesity and encourages it. Let's review some highlights of this crazy culture:

Super-Size Me

A traditional burger, fries and soft drink at a fast food restaurant used to contain over six hundred calories and almost twenty grams of fat. Today, the standard combo (with a large order of fries, double cheeseburger and large drink) has 1,805 calories and 84 grams of fat—nearly triple the calories and more than quadruple the fat! A standard serving of carbonated soda used to be 6.5 oz.—approximately ninety calories. Today, the standard serving is 20 oz. and packs 250 calories. There used to be only one size of a popular candy bar: 1.1 oz. or 210 calories. Today, the large size bar—3.7 oz.—more than doubles that with 500 calories.

Why have portions been super-sized? Like all companies, food and beverage companies—packaged goods and restaurants alike—aim to maximize their profits. And over the past generation, they realized that they can make more money through larger portions. If you're a fast food restaurateur and you charge $1.19 for a small fries and $1.79 for a large fries, on which item will you make the most money? The large fries, versus the small, includes a slightly larger box and the additional potatoes and oil. Those elements probably cost the owner just pennies per serving more than the small fries. Yet, you charge the customers an extra sixty cents; that could be almost pure profit. The overhead (the physical restaurant itself), the franchise fee, the labor, electricity—all these costs are the same regardless of whether the customer buys a small or a large. So, if you're the restaurant owner, your profit goes way up when you sell super-sized portions. Unfortunately, many people seem to value more food for their dollar, viewing it as a good deal. In fact, the company benefits from this good deal substantially. It's a bad deal for us.

Out to Lunch

With our fast-paced lifestyle, we're also eating more and more meals away from home, prepared by someone else. In 1975, Americans ate 25 percent of their meals outside of the home. In 2014, Americans will probably eat out for nearly 50 percent of their meals. Restaurant meals account for about fifty cents out of every dollar Americans spend on food—almost half of which is spent at fast-food eateries.

Eating out is convenient. It's fun. But the trade-off is control. By going out to eat, we're giving up control of ingredients, method of preparation and portion size. Because very few restaurants put your weight and health at the top of their agenda, you make compromises on each of these dimensions when you eat out. You would not make those compromises if you ate at home and retained control.

Advertising

Food and beverage companies try to generate good returns for their shareholders. It turns out that a good way to do that has been to market large portions of high-fat, calorie-dense foods to us and our children. Food and beverage marketers spend over fifteen billion dollars per year in the United States and Canada promoting their products to children and teens. Most of these ads show well-named junk food in colorful packaging that appeals quite a lot to children. And it works. Multiple studies have shown that children who are exposed to advertising ask their parents to buy high-fat, calorie-dense foods and sugary beverages. It's what kids want. It's what they pester you to buy. It's what they buy themselves. In their remarkable book *Food Fight*, Drs. Kelly Brownell and Katherine Horgen of Yale University pointed out a basic inequity: "At its peak, the 5-A-Day fruit and vegetable program from the National Cancer Institute had $2 million for promotion. This is one-fifth the $10 million used annually to advertise Altoids mints."

It's simply not a level playing field.

Advertising for soft drinks in the US has increased much faster in recent years than other advertising, going from $541 million in 1995 to $800 million in 1999—an almost 50 percent increase in four years. In the past generation, the percentage of American children who drink soda increased from 37 percent to over 60 percent, and average daily consumption among children who drink soda increased from 14 to 21 ounces. Researchers correlated amount of exposure to ads with a reduction in consumption of fruits and vegetables, presumably corresponding to an increase in the consumption of less nutritious foods. Every additional hour of television per day results in one less serving of fruits and vegetables every six days.

School Daze

Another important factor is the near elimination of physical education in most school districts. Forced to focus on reading and math test scores by federal and state governments, but with no more time and fewer resources, school officials cut electives like art, music and physical education. Today, only 8 percent of American elementary schools, 6 percent of middle schools and 5 percent of high schools provide daily physical education.

New World Living

In the US and Canada, 10 percent of city travel occurs outside of cars, buses or trains. In relatively newer cities, like Los Angeles, Atlanta and Dallas, where people rely on cars for almost everything, fewer than 5 percent of trips involve biking or walking. In contrast, people bike or walk to travel at least 40 percent in urban areas of Austria, Denmark, the Netherlands and Sweden. People travel by bike or walk for at least 30 percent of their urban trips in France, Germany and Switzerland.

Some of this change is due to the country where we're living. More Americans and Canadians now live in suburbs and so-called "exurbs" than ever before. Between 1970 and 2000, the percentage of Americans living in suburbs or exurbs grew from 38 percent to 50 percent. In the past fifty years, suburbs accounted for 90 percent of the growth in US metropolitan areas. People drive far more in such areas and builders no longer even lay down sidewalks where people live.

Suburban and exurban living has its benefits, but physical activity isn't one of them. Suburban dwellers weigh an average six pounds more than those who live in cities. Researchers have also connected time spent driving with obesity—the odds of being obese increase 6 percent with each hour per day spent in the car.

Being Sane in Insane Places

This phrase captures the quest for healthy living in modern, developed cultures. We get bombarded with ways of eating too much of the wrong kind of food and with appealing sedentary activities. Every new electronic gadget filled with apps enables us to do more by moving less. Every party and celebration includes so many caloric excesses that it becomes difficult to navigate life without developing excess weight. Currently, obesogenic culture wins far more than it loses.

OTHER CAUSAL ELEMENTS: BIOLOGY, PSYCHOLOGY, FAMILY AND EDUCATION

Figure 4-3 illustrates something that may seem surprising after reading about the power and pervasiveness of the obesogenic environment. This figure shows my perception of the relative importance of five causes of obesity. Notice the huge size of the biological slice of the pie. You will read a good deal about the major biological influences on weight in later chapters. Genetics play a major role in causing weight problems, but a dozen other biological forces impact tendencies to gain and lose excess weight (e.g., hormones, fat cells). Some people are born with a much greater propensity to gain weight and everyone who becomes overweight must overcome biological resistance that seems dead set on maintaining excess weight. Of course, athletes must overcome biological resistance, too. Overweight people have bodies that do not want to lose weight; athletes have bodies that do not want to train hard enough to master their sports. Both weight controllers and athletes, however, can learn how to overcome such barriers.

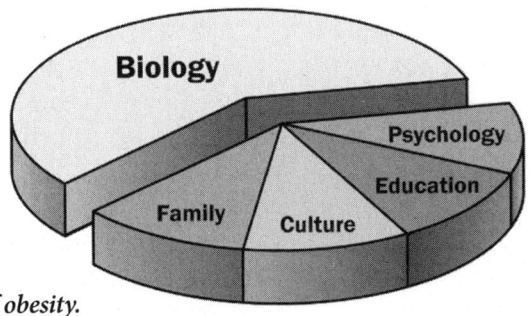

Figure 4-3. Five causes of obesity.

Biology Is Not Destiny.

The term *psychology* in the five causes illustration pertains to the intrapersonal factor described previously. That discussion mentioned that conscientiousness can help weight controllers and, conversely, emotional instability can interfere with success. Families that support their weight controllers also can help weight controllers succeed. If families become more active and embrace a very low-fat approach to eating, for example, research shows that their overweight young people succeed at much higher rates than those with less involved families. Finally, most people benefit from education about weight control, knowing what to do and how to do it. That includes recipes and also relevant information about diet and activities.

"Knowledge is power" works the other way too. Without knowing the best approach, many weight controllers get influenced by aggressive marketing to believe that some products can help them when they can't.

FIXES

Knowing the causes of weight problems provides some strong suggestions about likely fixes. If a proposed approach ignores the biology of weight gain, then it may not help you manage that key aspect of the challenge. Understanding our obesogenic culture and the insanity of it can prepare you for the battles ahead. The five causes shown in Figure 4-3 suggest that approaches to lose weight and keep it off must prepare weight controllers in comprehensive ways. All of the influences can make success either harder or easier depending on the approach.

In two recent papers that Kristen Gierut and I published, we reviewed five sets of recommendations published by groups of experts on how to treat childhood and adolescent obesity. The types of treatments that the expert groups considered for young people actually apply to people of all ages. Figure 4-4 illustrates the major options.

The box on the left side of Figure 4-4 indicates that Kristen Gierut and I described healthcare providers as sources of medical management and basic information of relevance to weight controllers. Medical management includes assessment of weight status and potential complications associated with excess weight, such as high blood pressure, high cholesterol levels and diabetes. Healthcare providers can also provide scientifically-based books and other materials, as well as make referrals to local specialists. Note the dashed line between the healthcare provider box and actual client behaviors/biology. This means that such medical management and educational information rarely produce changes in weight status (a biological function) or lifestyle behaviors. Referrals to specialists, however, can lead to major changes, as indicated by the solid lines between types of specialized interventions and changes in biology and behaviors.

Let's consider in more detail the five primary fixes for weight problems, starting with education. I'm not including medications in this list of potential fixes. The evidence just does not support the value of current medications for helping overweight people lose substantial amounts of weight in the long run. For example, one FDA-approved medication extracts fat from food that people eat, essentially helping them consume less fat. But that extracted fat causes many very unpleasant side effects, including occasionally uncontrollable bowel movements. Also, it seems better to follow a very low-fat diet instead of using this medication to produce a similar effect so unnaturally.

Education

The dashed arrow in Figure 4-4 from the healthcare provider box to client behaviors suggests that education alone usually fails to help people lose weight. Just telling people what to do simply does not help them do it very well. For example, Eric Stice and his colleagues provided the first

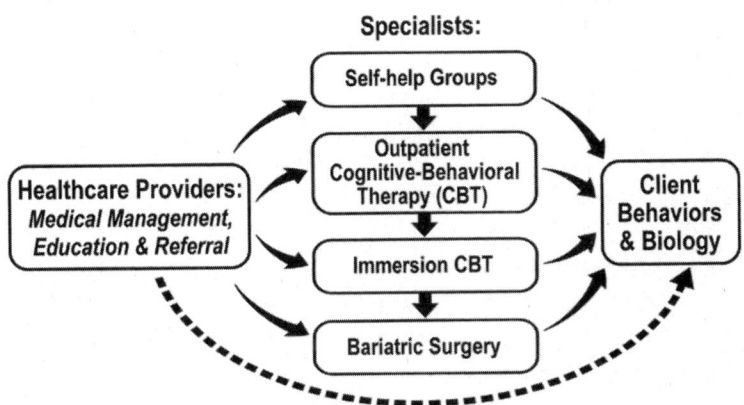

Figure 4-4. Treatment options for weight management and the process flowing from healthcare providers to specialists to clients.

comprehensive review of the effects of educational interventions designed to decrease Body Mass Indexes (BMI) in young people. Although most of the sixty-four programs reviewed lasted six months or longer, only 21 percent produced statistically reliable reductions in BMI. The reviewers described the average effects of these programs as so small that it "would be considered trivial by most researchers and clinicians." Only three programs—5 percent of those evaluated—produced significant effects that persisted over time.

Self-Help Groups

Successful weight controllers often report valuing ongoing support to help them succeed. Many studies show beneficial effects from sustained contact, including participation in self-help support groups. These findings support the value of what has been called a "Continuing Care Model" for the treatment of the chronic disease of obesity. For example, a randomized trial of the most widely used approach to self-help groups (Weight Watchers), found that, on average, participants in Weight Watchers lost 3.2 percent of their initial weight. Even this modest average weight loss was substantially better than those who received similar information but didn't attend groups (0 percent sustained weight reduction on average).

Outpatient Cognitive-Behavioral Therapy (CBT)

Outpatient CBT programs help people stay focused by encouraging self-monitoring—the writing down of details such as number of fat grams consumed every day. These programs also involve weekly goal setting, planning, problem solving and mastering stress management skills. Figure 4-5 summarizes some of these CBT techniques, among others.

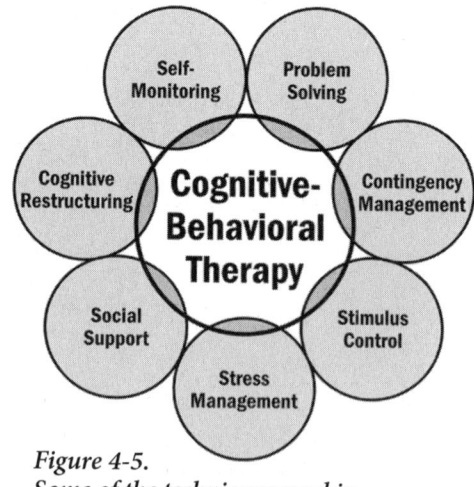

Figure 4-5.
Some of the techniques used in cognitive-behavioral therapy (CBT).

Studies show that people do lose meaningful amounts of weight in such programs and keep the weight off, in many cases for years. However, this doesn't happen for most participants, especially those who do not stay involved for at least several months.

Factors that contribute to the variability of the outcomes in outpatient CBT approaches include the practical challenges involved with just showing up every week. It's hard to make time in a busy life to go to a meeting, usually in the evenings, every single week. Also, weight loss varies a lot in such programs. During some weeks people gain weight; in other weeks they lose. In a recent paper, Joseph Skelton and his colleagues reviewed rates of attrition in such outpatient CBT clinics. These authors reported an average attrition of 54 percent across five large-scale clinics, including their own. That means more than half of the people who start out in these programs drop out after only a few weeks. That does not provide continuing care at all, regardless of the quality of the programs.

Immersion CBT

Immersion treatment places overweight people in a therapeutic and educational environment for extended periods of time, thereby removing them from obesogenic surroundings. In contrast to outpatient treatment, immersion treatments (those involving at least ten consecutive days and nights of participation) are more easily accessed by people from diverse locations. Immersion also minimizes the attrition problem that clearly limits the potential impact of outpatient treatment.

Immersion treatments for young people and adults have produced promising results. Kristina Pecora Kelly and I provided the first comprehensive review of this research, involving twenty-two outcome studies. We concluded that "Compared to results highlighted in a recent meta-analysis of outpatient treatments, these immersion programs produced an average of 197 percent greater reductions in percent-overweight at post-treatment and 130 percent greater reduction at follow-up. Furthermore, mean attrition rates were much lower when compared to standard outpatient treatment. Inclusion of a CBT component seems especially promising; follow-up evaluations showed decreased percent-overweight at follow-up by an average of 30 percent for CBT immersion programs versus 9 percent for programs without CBT."

I proposed the Immersion-to-Lifestyle Change model as an explanation for the promising results obtained in CBT immersion treatments. As

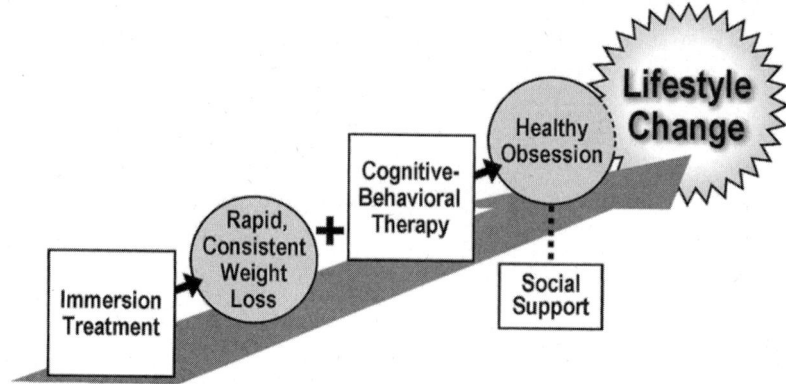

Figure 4-6. The Immersion-to-Lifestyle Change Model.

shown in Figure 4-6, this model suggests that rapid weight loss combined with CBT may help weight controllers attribute their successes to their own efforts. This, in turn, could increase self-efficacy (self-confidence), reinforce skills like goal setting and self-monitoring and maximize commitment. The culmination of these effects, in combination with social support, might enhance healthy obsessions. A healthy obsession is the consistent preoccupation with planning and executing target behaviors to reach a healthy goal. This type of intensive focusing seems necessary for success in weight control.

Bariatric Surgery

I believe bariatric surgery (a variety of procedures including gastric bands and bypasses) holds some promise, but this extreme intervention quite often creates troublesome side effects and is only available for limited numbers of extremely overweight people. Many very overweight people do benefit from this major procedure, but most overweight and obese people would find their lives disrupted less by using the Wellspring Plan and some of the interventions described in this chapter to succeed instead.

SUMMARY

Table 4-1 summarizes the effects of the five approaches to fix weight problems considered in this chapter. As you can see, education rarely seems to produce benefits in the long run by itself. In combination with outpatient

Table 4-1
Effectiveness of Five Approaches to Weight Management

Education	• Minimal effects • 5% may benefit significantly
Self-Help	• 20–50% may benefit long-term
Outpatient Cognitive-Behavioral Therapy	• 20% may benefit long-term
Bariatric Surgery	• 33–50% show substantial improvement, but available for limited population • Some post-surgical complications
Immersion CBT Programs	• Good potential for long-term change • 33–50% may benefit long-term

CBT or self-help, quite a few people can improve their health and happiness, grounded in useful knowledge. Bariatric surgery may produce substantial improvements for extremely overweight people, but it comes with sometimes significant financial and physical costs. Finally, immersion CBT seems quite promising for those who can afford such programs.

Figure 4-7 summarizes the key elements of Wellspring's version of an immersion CBT program. For those who cannot afford the more

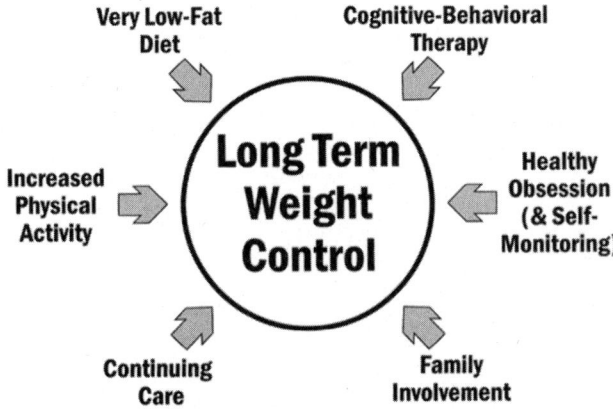

Figure 4-7. Elements of Wellspring's Immersion CBT Program.

expensive approaches, good self-help programs may prove quite useful. That comes closest to providing the continuing care and focusing that many people find helpful. For all weight controllers, obtaining a thorough knowledge of what helps and what doesn't provides the foundation for change. The next seven chapters will describe the seven steps of the Wellspring Plan and hopefully refine your understanding of what it takes to succeed as a weight controller-athlete.

PART 3

Wellspring's Seven Steps to Become a Weight Controller-Athlete

CHAPTER 5

Step 1—Understand Your Body's Resistance to Weight Loss

When my colleagues and I created Wellspring in 2004 we began with a trio of concepts that we believed would make weight loss most successful: simple, scientific and sustainable. By "simple" we meant easily remembered, clear and measurable—not easy. "Scientific" meant that we wanted to rely on principles demonstrated through science as much as possible to create all aspects of the program, from eating to activities to lifestyle change. Finally, "sustainable" referred to the ultimate goal, to create a program that did not just help people lose weight initially, but instead helped them sustain weight changes for the rest of their lives.

This thinking led to the creation of a version of the 3-1-7 program, which conveys three simple goals, one overarching mission and seven steps to get there. The three simple goals summarize three of the most important and easily remembered goals of the Wellspring Plan. The overarching mission, to develop a healthy obsession, captures the single most important goal in the program. *A healthy obsession is the preoccupation with planning and executing target behaviors to reach a healthy goal.* That type of intensive focus seems necessary for effective weight control, especially in the long run. Finally, the steps necessary to reach the three simple goals and the overarching mission include understanding the biological challenge and learning other key things to help reach the goals most consistently and comfortably. In this chapter we'll focus on understanding these concepts and techniques so you can use them to nurture your own weight controller-athlete.

3 Simple Behavioral Goals	• Eat 0g fat daily (accept 20g) • Get 12,000 steps per day • Self-monitoring 100 percent
1 Overarching Mission	To Develop a Healthy Obsession
7 Steps	1. Understand Your Body's Resistance to Weight Loss 2. Create a Powerful Commitment to Succeed 3. Manage Food to Lose Weight Most Comfortably 4. Use Movement to Level the Playing Field 5. Develop an Athlete's Healthy Obsession 6. Build a Winning Team Around You 7. Become Undisturbable

What makes losing weight and keeping it off so difficult?

Most people answer this question by invoking challenges like fast food, instant messaging, super-sized portions and busy lifestyles. Although these factors certainly contribute to the problem, what is the chief culprit? If you had to pick one primary factor that causes weight problems more than any other, what would you say? More specifically, answer the second part of this question: What makes losing weight and keeping it off so difficult? Is it biology or everything else?

By biology, we mean genes (inherited tendencies), fat cells, hormones, enzymes and metabolic rates (the amount of energy your body requires to simply stay alive at rest). "Everything else" refers to culture, family influences, habits, lifestyles, personality and emotional functioning. Both biology and everything else clearly influence weight. But, if you had to pick one as your primary culprit which one would you select? Does biology or everything else have the most powerful impact on your weight?

If you answered like 95 percent of people to whom I've posed this question, you would say that both answers were correct, but that "everything else" clearly has the edge over "biology." This is the logical answer. After all, the environment, culture, our habits and lifestyle seem to be responsible for weight gain. However, that perfectly logical and reasonable answer isn't the best one.

Biology makes losing weight and keeping it off extremely difficult, even more so than "everything else." The result of research by Canadian psychologist Claude Bouchard at Laval University made this point. Dr. Bouchard and his colleagues studied twelve sets of young male identical twins who lived in a controlled environment for one hundred days. After a baseline period of twelve days, the twins were given 1,000 calories above their usual levels of intake for the next eighty-four days. Some participants gained about nine pounds but others gained almost thirty pounds—all under virtually identical conditions. The best predictor of how much weight any one boy gained was how much his twin gained. Some twins apparently had the biological tendency to gain weight easily, whereas others did not.

If you fully understand the power of biology as a cause of this problem, you will appreciate why becoming a successful weight controller demands considerable effort and support. Weight controllers have to learn what is and what isn't okay for them at home and when eating out. In sharp contrast, those who do not have this biological handicap don't ever have to think about it.

Developing an understanding of these biological challenges can help you start down the path of long-term weight control. This understanding begins by considering the biological demands faced by our collective ancestors.

OUR HUNTER-GATHERER BODIES

Let's take an imaginary trip back in time. Experts tell us that somewhere between seven to ten thousand years ago humans began farming, raising crops and keeping animals. Try to imagine what life was like in the two hundred to three hundred thousand years before that happened, when the first people who had bodies very much like ours were born.

- We would wake up in a different place every day because, without domestic animals or crops, we had to search for food.
- We would be members of a tribe of ten to twenty people, depending on each other for survival.
- We would all be focused on four goals: find food, find shelter, raise our families and most of all, stay alive.
- Look around at your fellow tribe members. Everyone would be muscular from years of hard work. Exercise was a foreign concept

because staying alive required moving, hunting, fishing, foraging and avoiding danger ten to fifteen hours a day. Those who were not agile simply wouldn't survive. The best of the best of us survived and passed those traits down to our children.

- It's been several days with very little food. The dried meat ran out three days ago. Driven by a deep hunger, you search frantically for food. Along the way you find a few berries in the melting spring snow, but it doesn't do much for that gnawing sensation in the pit of your stomach.
- Up ahead, you hear the hunters shouting with excitement as they corner a young deer. With skill in throwing primitive spears and rocks, a little luck and a powerful desire to survive, they bring the deer down to the ground. Everyone cheers because tonight, you will have food! It also means you can rest tomorrow, because you don't have to hunt. You can set up a base camp and dry and tan the deer's hide, dry pieces of the meat and take stock of how you're doing. That's a good thing, because you probably took 50,000 steps today.
- Think of how you'll eat the deer meat. Will you eat it slowly, savoring each bite? Or will you gobble it down? Because you're starving and because if you don't someone else will, you'll eat it as quickly as you can.

Fast forward a few hundred thousand years:

- You now have a small farm and some animals fenced in.
- You don't have to get up every day and go out searching for food.
- With all this additional time, you can improve your tools, create art and music and, unfortunately, invent ways to take over other tribes.
- Still, you end up spending many hours a day doing physical labor and grappling with the inevitable famines that occur about every two years. You average 30,000 steps every day.

Fast forward to today:

- You drive to work.
- You sit at a desk and talk to people on the phone or in meetings.

- You pick up lunch at the drive-thru and gobble it down.
- You return to work.
- You drive home.
- You eat dinner, read and watch television.
- Your pedometer registers only 4,000 steps today—about average for Americans.

You probably understand the huge problem we all face: Our bodies still "think" we are all hunter-gatherers, storing fat efficiently and resisting weight loss aggressively to safeguard against famines of short and long duration. Also, our bodies were designed to move—to move a lot—for most of the day. In the few remaining countries and cultures where people still move around a great deal throughout the day, weight problems remain relatively rare. By contrast, modern American culture encourages very sedentary living. A majority of American adults are now overweight at least in part because they don't move around enough. Finally, the same biological forces that caused you to quickly gobble up the deer meat are also creating the impulse to gulp down lunch at the drive-thru.

It's a wonder everyone isn't overweight. Why do some people remain thin despite these powerful forces?

Undoubtedly you know people who seem to eat anything and everything, probably far more than you do, yet remain thin. Our sedentary culture and abundance of foods affects some people far more than others. Some people inherit the tendency to gain weight easily, whereas some inherit the tendency to stay slim. Others who gain weight in middle age, unfortunately, develop those biological tendencies to promote weight gain and resist weight loss later in life. These biological factors have a pronounced impact on weight.

BIOLOGICAL BARRIERS TO WEIGHT LOSS

Let's consider some of the details of these biological barriers to help you appreciate and accept their power. Just remember one critical caveat as you read about them:

Biology Is Not Destiny.

If biology were fully and completely in charge, no one would ever lose weight and keep it off. Biology makes it tough for athletes to develop the speed, strength and skills they strive to achieve. Athletes learn how to manage those biological resistances; so do successful weight controllers.

There are actually twelve distinct biological factors that make weight control quite difficult. Whenever people develop excess weight (at any point in their lives) their bodies become especially efficient and effective at maintaining higher-than-normal levels of fat. These biological forces include ones that begin their work before a baby takes its first breath and others that develop over the years. Five of these biological factors are especially impressive and memorable—and may help remind you of the power of this biological foe.

1. Genes

Genetic factors are those that are inherited from our parents and prior generations. In breeding studies with mice, fatter mice have been mated with other fatter mice and leaner mice with other leaner mice. Over fifteen to twenty-five generations, this can produce mice pups from the fatter matings with twice as much fat as the pups from the leaner matings. This research shows the tremendous degree to which inheritance of genetic makeup determines the tendency to develop excess fat.

Human parallels include research showing that children born to parents who are both obese are four times more likely to become obese than children born to lean parents. Some recent research on twins also emphasizes the degree to which inheritance plays a role in developing excess weight. A study by Dr. Claude Bouchard in Canada involved overfeeding twelve pairs of identical twins for one hundred days. If one member of a twin pair gained a lot of weight, the other member of the pair did also. In addition, the twins who gained more weight tended to gain more of the weight as fat and less of it as lean body tissues (such as muscles or organs).

Other studies with twins growing up in separate households have shown similar trends: the twin siblings resembled each other in weight status much more than other siblings with whom they grew up. These findings show that some of us are born with bodies primed to gain weight easily from day one while others may resist weight gain. Just as genetics dramatically affect weight gain, it similarly affects weight regain after losing it.

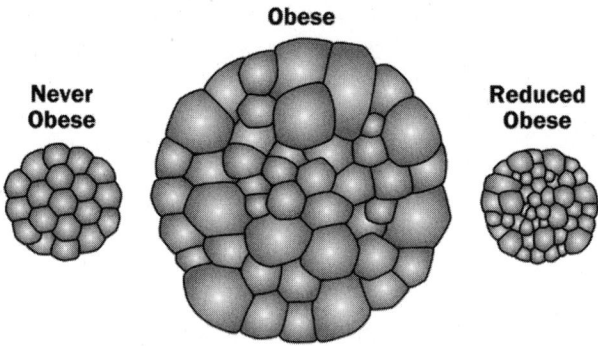

2. Fat Cells = Hungry Baby Sparrows

Beyond genetics, overweight people have many more fat cells than people who have never been overweight. How many more? Overweight people can have *four times* as many of these hungry creatures (e.g., one hundred and sixty billion versus forty billion). Your fat cells act like hungry baby sparrows, with their mouths wide open looking for more food. Unfortunately, liposuction can only remove a few million of these—barely making a dent because fat is intertwined in our muscles and organs. You can also develop more fat cells at any point in your life. And it doesn't take long to add fat cells. Some studies have shown that animals that are fed large amounts of high-fat food can permanently gain excess fat cells within one week.

Most critically, once fat cells develop, they never disappear. Why is this so important? The importance comes from the fact that fat cells promote very efficient storage of excess food as fat. Studies have traced where the body sends fat after eating. For overweight and formerly overweight people, the body delivers fat into the fat cells more efficiently (perhaps directed by some of the biological devices described below). People who have never had weight problems seem to have more fat transported into muscles for use as immediate fuel. The next figure illustrates these differences in fat cells, before and after weight loss.

3. Hormones and Enzymes.

There are a number of hormones and enzymes that evolution has established as biological barriers against weight loss. While it's not essential that you understand the mechanics of each one, the overall picture is daunting. We'll walk through them one by one to give you a sense of what you're up against.

Insulin

The concentration of blood sugar (glucose) in our bodies is regulated very carefully in people who are not diabetic. The body must maintain this regulation because the brain depends totally on blood sugar for its nutrition. And if our brains aren't properly nourished, we can't survive. This regulation is keyed by a detector in the brain that determines when blood sugar levels are too high or too low. Insulin, which is stored and manufactured in special cells within the pancreas, promotes the ingestion of glucose by our cells.

When people lose weight, the body's fat cells become especially sensitive to insulin. That enables the cells to absorb more nutrients at a faster pace. The muscle cells decrease their sensitivity to insulin, resulting in redirection of fat to the fat cells. Several studies have shown that some people develop an especially high level of insulin sensitivity when they lose weight; these people tend to regain weight very readily. It seems that a great many overweight people are quite sensitive to insulin and can very quickly store excess nutrients as fat partly because of this tendency. Most overweight people also have excessive amounts of insulin in their blood stream at all times, which may contribute to the efficiency with which their bodies become sensitive to insulin as they lose weight.

LPL

Lipoprotein lipase (LPL) is an enzyme (special chemical agent) produced in many cells. It stays on the walls of very small blood vessels and can become activated to transport fat in the body. During weight loss, increases in LPL occur as fat cells release their LPL into the bloodstream. By doing so, the fat cells send messages to the brain: "Get more food in us, now!"

Perhaps part of this drive to eat came from attempts to decrease eating occasionally. Biologically, this means that weight loss stimulated hunger and helped convert food into stored fat. At least for some people, LPL activity is especially high and probably makes it more difficult for them to maintain weight loss.

Leptin

Leptin, a hormone discovered in 1994, is secreted by fat cells to act as a messenger between the cells and the brain, directing the amount of fat that gets stored in fat cells by affecting appetite. As the fat cells expand during weight gain, leptin is released by those cells. Increasing circulating levels of leptin can decrease appetite and in turn contribute to maintenance of healthy weights; conversely, problems with recognition of leptin in the brain (receptors in the hypothalamus) may increase excess weight.

Ghrelin

The hormone ghrelin is one of the strongest appetite stimulants known. It is produced in the stomach, which releases more ghrelin as people lose weight. For example, one study found that when weight controllers lost 17 percent of their body weight, their levels of ghrelin rose by 24 percent. Further substantiating the importance of ghrelin, weight loss surgery (such as the gastric bypass) decreases ghrelin substantially. With less appetite (due to decreased ghrelin), those who undergo these surgeries don't have to fight the ghrelin battle.

Adiponectin

Adiponectin is a protein secreted by fat cells (like leptin) that helps insulin direct blood sugar from the blood stream into your body's cells. When blood sugar goes into your cells it is stored or burned for fuel in those cells. Unfortunately, the more fat cells and larger fat cells a person has, the less adiponectin the fat cells secrete. This effect of adiponectin means that overweight people have a greater propensity to direct blood sugar into fat cells rather than using it for energy.

Because of adiponectin, ghrelin, leptin, LPL and insulin, the body powerfully resists weight loss for overweight people.

4. Adaptive Thermogenesis.

When weight controllers attempt to lose weight and reduce the amount of food they consume, their bodies have the capability to switch into a very efficient mode. Remember the plight of the hunter-gatherers, whose bodies we have inherited. In order for them to survive, their bodies had to make adjustments when they couldn't catch a deer in a particular week. Adaptive thermogenesis allowed their bodies to survive on fewer calories (greater efficiency, slower metabolism) during times when adequate amounts of food simply weren't available.

This means that reducing calorie intake by, say, five hundred calories a day may not promote any weight loss if the weight controller's body uses adaptive thermogenesis to switch from its normal mode to a much more efficient mode. The good news about adaptive thermogenesis is that you can reverse this effect by moving more than usual or exercising every day. This exercise effect makes it possible for weight controllers to lose weight by bypassing the effects of adaptive thermogenesis (remaining in the relatively inefficient mode that burns more calories).

5. Set-point

As a weight controller tries to lose weight, his or her body uses adaptive thermogenesis to become efficient. The body also relies on its use of various hormones and enzymes (like insulin, leptin, LPL), to make it difficult to lose weight and keep it off. The fat cells themselves, including their unusual ability to expand in size and number, also contribute to this problem. The set-point concept summarizes all of these effects, making it clear that weight controllers are stuck in bodies that utilize a variety of biological forces to resist weight loss. Just as leptin has been a recent discovery, undoubtedly there are other biological mechanisms that contribute to the body's desire to maintain an excessive amount of fat. Research with animals has shown that very overweight rats and mice show similar tendencies to "defend" (or "set") the amount of fat in their bodies at a very high level.

Unfortunately, part of this defense (or set-point) includes a tendency for the body of overweight people to respond more dramatically to the sight, smell and even the thought of tempting foods. A study by psychologists William Johnson and Hal Wildman at the University of Mississippi Medical School confirmed this. These researchers showed that overweight participants, compared to their lean counterparts, increased their insulin responses not only to the actual sight and smell of bacon and eggs, but to the thought of bacon and eggs. The overweight participants also salivated more when they saw or thought about tasty foods. This means that overweight people may defend their high weights by over-secreting insulin and digestive enzymes. These biological responses can increase the desire to consume more food in order to decrease the levels of these substances in the bloodstream.

ACCEPTING THE BIOLOGICAL REALITY

These biological factors create real and powerful resistance to weight loss for you. It's not simply a question of your willpower. You face definite biological challenges that require minimizing and managing. There is no escaping this reality. When you think about it, the biology of obesity makes a lot of sense. Why would so many people have so much difficulty maintaining weight loss if biological forces did not resist weight loss? Losing weight produces many positive rewards, but relatively brief lapses in concentration (for example, occasional overeating of high-fat foods and inconsistent exercising) are eagerly greeted by your body's extra billions of fat cells. That's a lot of hungry sparrows to feed! These fat cells and other biological forces are always present, ready to pounce.

The good news here is that once you accept the powerful role that biology plays in creating and maintaining weight problems, you can deflect some of the blame and shame away from your personality or basic self. Weight control is not a question of changing from an abnormal state of gluttony to a normal state of controlled eating. You must change from a relatively normal state of functioning with an unfortunate biology to a set of behaviors that must be considered super-normal (i.e., beyond the norm, or extraordinary). This makes weight control one of the most difficult challenges a person can face.

Just remember the caveat at the beginning of this chapter: **Biology is not destiny.** Athletes overcome the resistance of their bodies; so do successful weight controllers.

CHAPTER 6

Step 2—Develop a Powerful Commitment to Change

While it's true that the benefits of weight loss dramatically outweigh the costs required to change, this is only true if you utilize an approach that can really help you succeed. One of the major obstacles to establishing a desire to change is that many overweight children, teens and adults don't believe that anything can help them succeed. They have been trying diet after diet, losing some weight, regaining it and then gaining more. Most weight controllers have spent the better part of their lives failing at this very important aspect of their existence.

ALL PERSONAL CHANGES ARE CHALLENGING

In their fascinating book *Facilitating Treatment Adherence*, Canadian psychologists Don Meichenbaum and Dennis Turk describe a remarkable example of how people resist change, despite sometimes dire consequences. Patients who were diagnosed with glaucoma—a serious, but treatable disease of the eye—were told that "they must use eye drops three times per day or they would go blind." The study revealed that only 42 percent of patients used the eye drops as instructed. Remarkably, a majority failed to follow the regimen carefully enough to avoid permanent damage to their eyes. Even after becoming legally blind in one eye, only 28 percent changed course and began following the instructions more carefully.

Newton's first law of physics is inertia. Inertia means that objects don't move unless they're forced to move. People are the same as objects in this respect. We resist change mightily. Consider some additional statistics cited by Meichenbaum and Turk, about the extent to which we resist change:

- **Prescriptions.** Approximately one-third of the 750 million new prescriptions written annually in the United States and England are never filled. Also, the directions of 300 million new prescriptions are not followed in the way they are written.
- **Adolescent cancer.** Approximately 50 percent of medications prescribed to adolescents with cancer are not taken as directed.
- **Epilepsy.** Approximately 35 percent of the drug regimens prescribed for epilepsy are not followed.
- **Pediatric illness.** Parents fail to ensure that their children adhere to medication regimens approximately 50 percent of the time.
- **Schizophrenia.** Approximately 75 percent of people diagnosed with schizophrenia discontinue treatment prematurely.
- **Chronic illness among the elderly.** A majority of elderly people who have chronic illnesses do not follow their prescribed and necessary medication regimens.
- **Kidney disease.** Approximately 70 percent of people with kidney disease fail to follow dietary and fluid restrictions necessary for their comfort and health.
- **High blood pressure.** Only 30 percent of people with high blood pressure follow the medical regimens that can save their lives.
- **Exercise.** Only 20 percent of adult Americans exercise at least twice a week for at least 30 minutes. The American College of Sports Medicine recommends that everyone should exercise at least five times per week.

These statistics are startling. You may wonder after reading this, "How could people fail to do what they need to do to stay healthy and alive?" The fact is that people usually struggle to maintain regimens of any kind that force them to behave differently from their usual routines.

Weight control is one of the greatest personal challenges that anyone can face and you may find yourself resisting changes in your own lifestyle and routines. In the next section, we'll review several decisional counseling techniques that can help you strengthen your commitment enough to battle this internal resistance to change. These procedures provide a framework for fleshing out the benefits and challenges and ultimately making the decision to pursue long-term weight control.

DECISIONAL COUNSELING TECHNIQUES

How committed are you to losing weight right now? Is it one of the top two or three priorities in your life at the moment? Does it fall somewhere much further down the list? Is it even on the list?

One way to ensure it's where it will do you some good (probably among the top two or three priorities) is to use decisional counseling. The principle is this: When you thoroughly analyze the possible advantages and disadvantages of a particular goal, you almost always become more committed to that goal. So by analyzing the possible advantages and disadvantages of pursuing long-term weight control, your commitment to pursuing this challenging goal can increase.

Create a Decision Balance Sheet

The box which follows will show you how to begin this process. Here's how to use this powerful tool:

1. Select a goal.

First, write in a specific goal for the next year. For example, are you going to lose twenty, fifty or one hundred pounds during this next year? When writing out the goal, consider that it works best to state a goal that is difficult but achievable. For most people, a realistic goal for weight loss at home is between ¼ and 1 lb. per week. If you don't know what seems reasonable as a goal for weight loss, visit the Centers for Disease Control's website and use their BMI calculator to determine your ideal weight.

2. Write out the pros and cons.

After stating your goal, write out everything you can think of that would be good or positive about reaching this goal. How would a twenty-pound weight loss impact your life?

After writing down the good things, consider the challenges. Weight control takes time, effort and money for everyone who seeks it.

Decision Balance Sheet

Name: _____ Date: _____

What I'm trying to change: _____

Good Things About Doing This	Challenging Things About Doing This
1. _____	1. _____
2. _____	2. _____
3. _____	3. _____
4. _____	4. _____
5. _____	5. _____
6. _____	6. _____
7. _____	7. _____
8. _____	8. _____

Decision Balance Sheet: EXAMPLE

Name: *Jane S.* Date: *3/3*

What I'm trying to change: **To lose 20 lbs.**

Good Things About Doing This	Challenging Things About Doing This
1. *Look better*	1. *I'd feel like a failure if I don't do it*
2. *Feel better about myself*	2. *It will be frustrating sometimes.*
3. *Get new clothes*	3. *Maybe I still won't look too good.*
4. *Get cuter clothes.*	4. *It will be hard work.*
5. *Fewer nasty comments*	5. *I might miss some foods.*
6. *Look more attractive to guys*	6. *Doing it will draw attention to me*
7. *Healthier*	7. *I'll get tired*
8. *Parents will be very proud*	

What are the specific costs of having your weight controller attempt to lose weight this year? Write out the challenges as well.

3. Review the example for additional ideas.

This example is compiled from decision balance sheets completed by many of the teenagers in Wellspring's programs. If you are seeking additional ideas, see if discussing each item with a trusted friend or family member helps you generate additional points for your decision balance sheet. The more factors you can include on both positive and negative sides, the better.

4. Reviewing and Rating

Review both columns carefully. Which is more compelling? It's not a simple count of pros versus cons. This exercise requires you to study the importance of each item on the list. It's often helpful to take time to rate the importance of each item. Use a 10 point scale in which 10 means "extremely important" and 1 means "not at all important." For Jane (the woman whose Decision Balance Sheet we just looked at), you can see that her challenges seem rather minor in most cases. For example, getting tired and feeling frustrated are temporary states and probably warrant low ratings. Also, you could argue—and we encourage you to do this with yourself—that feeling a little tired or frustrated sometimes pales in comparison to feeling so much better physically and emotionally in the long run.

5. Balance!

Review your ratings and discuss them with a friend, family member or therapist. See if you can come to some consensus about how to rate every item. If not, average your ratings, then put that average rating next to each item. Add up both columns. In most cases, the column for the good things clearly outweighs the challenges. If this isn't the case, you're going to have to work through a few more things or get additional help to get yourself there.

Reaffirm Your Commitment

The Decision Balance Sheet should remain an active part of your weight control process. Please keep it handy or make copies so you can review it over and over again. Another option is to re-rate both columns. This is typically quite energizing.

These techniques are particularly useful when the going gets a bit rough—for example, if you work hard at your program, but gain a half pound in a week. As you will learn in subsequent sections, every weight controller has setbacks. Reaffirming commitment by using the power of choice can be a useful technique.

HANG UP PICTURES THAT MOTIVATE

Some people carry pictures of themselves at either slimmer or heavier weights to motivate them. Other motivating images can be found by looking through magazines. Some weight controllers hang pictures or posters of activities like rafting or tennis, or even photos of clothes, to keep them focused. If you want to fit into an old outfit, consider hanging the outfit where it can be seen. At least one study has demonstrated tangible benefits from such imagery. Concentration boils down to thinking about something quite often. Images can be very useful in promoting this.

PREMACKING

"Premacking" (named for psychologist Dr. David Premack) involves reinforcing an unlikely behavior by pairing it with a likely behavior. You can write down several key words on the back of a business card and place the card in your wallet. For example:

- Acceptance
- Mastery
- Self-confidence
- Clothes
- Health
- Energy
- Looks

Reviewing these words regularly is an "unlikely behavior." Every time you use your wallet or perhaps every time you use either a debit or credit card (a "likely behavior"), you can take a few seconds to review the card. Each of the points on the card means something important about your commitment to weight control. So every time you review the card, spend a few seconds reflecting on the importance of weight control in your life (i.e., the good side of the Decision Balance Sheet). It just takes a few seconds to review these important goals. Premacking the value of feeling more energetic and looking good can get those positive expectations flowing more intensely.

CONCLUSION

We follow routines for complex reasons. Our genetics, history, traditions, personalities, preferences, demands from others and other factors determine how we spend every day. Making the changes required for weight loss produces an almost reflexive resistance. I hope that you understand these very common feelings and that you've managed to use the Decision Balance Sheet and other ideas in this chapter to help establish a stronger commitment to change.

CHAPTER 7

Step 3—Manage Food to Lose Weight Most Comfortably

The information in this chapter can help you tame those savage little beasts, those extra billions of fat cells that make their presence known to your appetite every day. Thousands of successful weight controllers have managed to satisfy these hungry sparrow-beasts; you can too.

In this chapter we'll focus on eight things that have the greatest effects on your hunger, weight and long-term prospects for success: fat, sugar, protein, energy density, fiber, caloric beverages, calorie consciousness and the lovability of your food. You will find the principles of eating that emerge from this review much more sensible but a bit more challenging than the ones in Table 7-1:

Table 7-1

Top 10 Rules for Easier Weight Control in a Saner, Fairer World

10. Food consumed for medicinal purposes doesn't have any calories. This includes throat lozenges, cough drops, chicken noodle soup and anything else bought in a Jewish deli.

9. Using sugar substitutes in coffee entitles you to a free dessert every once in a while. Every once in a while includes two Fridays on either side of your birthday and every Saturday night except for the second Saturday in February.

8. Snacks consumed after midnight don't count because "it could have been a dream, anyway."
7. Pieces of cookies, bagels and cheese (not cubes or slices) have no calories. The process of breaking uses more calories than the pieces contain.
6. If you drink a diet soda with pretzels or popcorn, the pretzels and popcorn have no calories. First of all, the pretzels and (low-fat) popcorn are healthy snacks, anyway. Second, the calories in these good snacks are canceled by the diet soda.
5. If you eat with someone else, the calories you consume don't count if you eat less than they do.
4. Foods that have the same color have the same number of calories, for example, tomato sauce and cherry pie, yogurt and cheesecake.
3. Tasting food while preparing it is not really eating. Licking peanut butter off the knife while making a sandwich for your son or daughter is necessary to ensure the adequacy of the peanut butter, and, therefore, no calories are consumed during this important parental task.
2. If you eat something very quickly and/or if no one sees you eat it, it has no calories. Maybe it never happened?
1. Snacks eaten at movies or theaters (for example, candy, buttered popcorn, chocolate bon-bons) have no calories because they are part of the entire entertainment experience.

The "Healthy Eating Basics" described next can help you develop a balanced, healthful foundation to your weight control efforts.

HEALTHY EATING BASICS: A BALANCED APPROACH

To encourage Americans to eat a varied and balanced diet, and thereby consume adequate amounts of vitamins, minerals and fiber, the US Department of Agriculture officially launched the Food Guide Pyramid in 1992. In 2011, the USDA replaced the pyramid with the "My Plate" icon, pictured. The USDA plate presents five food groups, with the grain group (bread, cereal, rice and pasta) and the vegetable group taking up most of the space.

The USDA website, myplate.gov, has tremendous amounts of information, available as videos, posters and tips of the day, among other things. These materials promote a balanced diet that would allow you to get all of the essential nutrients and vitamins. The following descriptions summarize their recommendations about the five food groups, with the recommended numbers of servings based on a 2000 calorie per day diet:

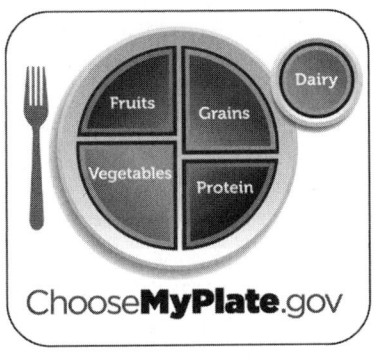

Vegetables: 2.5 cups per day

- 1 cup = a cup of raw or cooked vegetables; 2 cups of leafy salad vegetables = 1 cup of cooked vegetables
- Eat more red, orange and dark-green vegetables.
- Add beans or peas to salads, soups and side dishes.
- Fresh, frozen and canned vegetables all can work.

Fruits: 2 cups per day

- 1 cup = raw, cooked or 100 percent juice; ½ cup of dried fruit counts the same as 1 cup of raw fruit.
- Use fruits as snacks, salads and desserts.
- Top your cereal at breakfast with bananas or berries.

Grains: 6 ounces per day

- 1 ounce = 1 slice of bread, ½ cup cooked pasta, rice or cereal
- Substitute whole-grain choices for refined grains.
- Choose products that name a whole grain first on the ingredients list.

Dairy: 3 cups per day

- 1 cup = a cup of milk, yogurt or soymilk; 1.5 ounces natural cheese
- Choose skim or 1 percent milk.
- Top baked potatoes with low-fat yogurt.

Protein Foods: 5.5 ounces per day

- 1 ounce = 1 ounce of lean meat, poultry or fish; 1 egg; 1 Tbsn peanut butter; .5 oz nuts or seeds; .25 cup of beans or peas
- Eat a variety of foods from this group each week, such as seafood, beans and peas and nuts, as well as lean meats, poultry and eggs.
- Choose lean meats, trim or drain fat, have seafood twice a week.

If you follow the guidelines provided by My Plate, you probably will not benefit from taking vitamin or mineral supplements of any kind. However, because very few people follow this balanced approach, you would probably benefit from taking a multi-vitamin once per day. You can also see by the examples that many low-fat, low-calorie foods can be used to create a balanced meal plan. On the other hand, the plan you will find in the remainder of this chapter emphasizes an even lower-fat approach to eating.

Having an overall grasp of healthful, balanced eating provides the foundation for considering the eight keys to eating for weight loss. Please review those keys in Table 7-2 before beginning to read about the first key: very low-fat eating.

Table 7-2

Eight Keys to Eating to Lose Weight

1. Eat very little fat (aim for 0; less than 20g per day is okay).
2. Control your consumption of sugar.
3. Eat lean sources of protein frequently throughout the day, substituting plant for animal sources of protein as much as possible (70 g total protein; less than 30 g from animal sources).
4. Consume low-density foods (i.e., foods with few calories per gram of weight or ounce of volume).
5. Eat at least 30g of fiber per day.
6. Eat your calories—don't drink them.
7. Stay calorie conscious (e.g., maximum calories for biggest meal of the day = 800).
8. Find lovable foods that love you back.

GOOD-BYE FAT

"Any pig farmer knows that you can't get pigs fat feeding them wheat; you need corn, which contains more oil," says Professor Elliot Danforth. Danforth and his colleague Ethan Sims, both professors at the University of Vermont, studied the causes of obesity. Using male prisoners as subjects, they asked the prisoners to eat large amounts of food and then observed the effects. They found that the prisoners who ate a lot of high-fat foods gained much more weight than those who ate foods that were lower in fat and higher in carbohydrates.

High-fat foods are most easily stored as additional fat in the body. For example, to turn 100 calories of very high-fat foods like butter or bacon into body fat, your body only expends about three calories of energy. That means that ninety-seven of the 100 calories end up in your fat cells. Turning carbohydrates into fat is much more complicated. The body has to change the carbohydrate into a number of other chemical compounds in order to process it. As a result, in order to turn 100 calories of spaghetti into fat, the body has to expend about twenty-three calories. In other words, it costs very little energy to transform foods that already start out as fat into body fat. Therefore, 100 calories of spaghetti may translate into seventy-seven calories of fat, whereas 100 calories of butter transform into 97 calories of fat.

Your biology makes it especially easy for you to gain weight. Why make a bad situation worse by eating fat?

Fat Goal: How Low Can You Go?

In order to avoid eating fat, it helps to know how to measure the amount of fat in your diet. To do that it helps to buy a good calorie and fat gram counter, the best of which is the pocket-sized *The CalorieKing Calorie Fat and Carbohydrate Counter* by Allan Borushek (updated annually). CalorieKing also has a great website and app if you'd prefer a more high tech approach. Certain types of fat (like saturated fat, trans fat) create more cardiovascular health problems than other types of fat (for example, polyunsaturated fat, such as olive oil and peanut oil). However, successful weight controllers generally eat so little fat that they have to worry much less about which types of fat they consume than those who do not follow a very low-fat diet. From a weight control perspective:

A fat is a fat is a fat.

All fats contain approximately the same number of calories. Your body stores all fats very readily. In this respect:

*1 tablespoon of peanut oil = lard = corn oil = coconut oil = butter = **120 calories and 13.6 fat grams**.*

So, the question of greatest concern to those who want to lose weight is, "How little fat can I get myself to eat?" Do keep in mind, however, that plant sources of fat (like olive oil or canola oil) pose less danger for your long-term health than animal sources of fat (like butter or lard).

Some recent studies indicate that obese people eat higher percentages of their calories from fat than lean people. Most obese people eat similar numbers of total calories compared to non-obese individuals, but the percentages of fat in their diets can be 25 percent higher. If you want to lose weight, you must consume very little fat every day. The American Heart Association suggests that if Americans adopted a diet consisting of 30 percent of calories from fat, there would be much less heart disease in this country. Right now Americans consume closer to 34 percent of their total calories from fat. Reducing to diets containing 30 percent fat might improve the health of some people; but this level is still far too high for you and others who wish to lose weight. Some experts recommend that a better percentage for weight controllers is 20 percent. My recommendation is even simpler than that: consume as little fat as possible (and certainly less than 10 percent of all calories from fat)—and just add the total number of fat grams you consume each day, regardless of the percentage of calories from fat. So, the answer to the question, "How low can you go?" is: "As low as possible: **Aim for zero fat grams per day and accept no more than 20g.**" Not only is this "no fat" goal clearer than 10 percent or 20 percent of calories from fat, research suggests that it works better too.

Aim for Zero Fat Grams

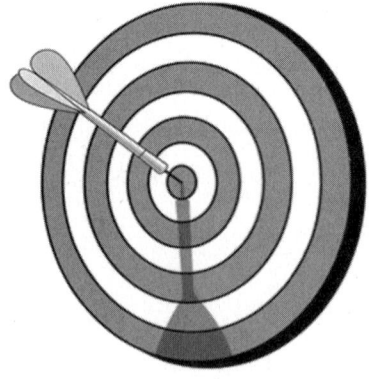

Living with such a very-low-fat eating plan presents challenges. This is the age of motorized dessert carts and specialty cookie shops seemingly on every street corner. While people talk about exercising more than ever before, many people exercise on their way to fast food restaurants. Who could forget the image of Bill Clinton jogging to a burger joint? Others enjoy wearing exercise clothes, but participating is a different story. The same applies to living life without high-fat foods. For example, in a recent *Consumer Reports* article entitled "Are You Eating Right?" the editors noted that Americans were "still saying 'cheese'." That is, "Americans have soured on whole milk in the past thirty years and now choose low-fat milk more often. But consumption of high-fat cheeses has more than doubled in the same period, and even cream is rising."

Virtually all successful weight controllers consume much less fat than do average Americans. This means that they rarely eat red meat, hardly ever eat desserts other than fruit or low-fat/no-fat alternatives and almost never eat fried foods. Their salad dressings are almost always fat-free, low-fat or low-calorie, and when they order salads in restaurants, salad dressings are ordered on the side. They grill, broil, bake and steam foods, and they insist on being served foods prepared in those low-fat ways in restaurants. Successful weight controllers rarely eat anything with high-fat gravies or sauces. No-fat or low-fat cheeses, ice cream and mayonnaises are also among their possibilities. They think of normal-fat cookies, brownies, cake and candy as foods for others, not for themselves.

Many people really *do* live this way (including me). For example, if you have made the change from whole milk to skim milk, do you miss drinking whole milk or does it seem more like cream to you now? People find some of these changes easier to implement than you might expect. For example, consider these comments from some of my more successful clients:

- "It's amazing, but I don't even want candy anymore. When I see candy, or people eating candy, I don't have the slightest interest in eating it."
- "I find fried foods disgustingly greasy now. Except for French fries, fried foods don't tempt me in the least. Okay, maybe onion rings tempt me a little, too."
- "This is the best time in history for living with fat-free and low-fat foods. There are so many perfectly good choices."
- "I now think of high-fat-foods as 'alien foods.' I say to myself, 'that stuff is for people from other worlds.'"

Fat-Free Eating Tips

Some ideas about food that have helped my clients make low-fat eating more palatable include ideas for making substitutions for high-fat foods, suggestions for staples in the cupboard and forty-two wonderful recipes in Part 4 of this book. Other ideas are:

- Snacks: air-popped popcorn, pretzels, fruit, rice cakes, sugar-free gelatin, low-calorie cocoa, the usual raw vegetables (pre-peeled mini-carrots and sugar snap peas are especially good)
- Mustard on everything: collect, compare and contrast many different varieties of mustards.
- Learn to love spicy foods.
- Salsa on everything: become a salsa connoisseur and collect, compare and contrast many different varieties.
- Pasta, pasta, pasta
- Tomato sauces: particularly low-fat versions
- Fish, shellfish
- Stir-fried cooking: use broths, water and no oil if possible.
- No-fat cheeses: try melting them on bagels or English muffins.
- Baked white or sweet potatoes with non-fat sour cream, cottage cheese or yogurt—Honey mustard works well too as a topping for potatoes.
- Soups: experiment with vegetables, beans and bones.
- Frozen entrees that specify amount of fat
- Canned, no-fat soups
- Use applesauce and new oil and shortening replacement products made of fruit purees instead of butter and oil in baked goods (see Part 4 of the book for the amounts to use based on the amounts of fat required in the recipe).
- Add fat-free broths, not oils, to marinades.
- Wrap fish in lettuce before baking to retain moisture. (Remove lettuce before serving—unless, of course, you love the taste of soggy, fishy lettuce!)
- To prevent yogurt from separating when heated, add one teaspoon of cornstarch for every cup of yogurt.

Step 3—Manage Food to Lose Weight Most Comfortably 121

- Use yogurt or evaporated skim milk or cottage cheese instead of cream.
- Vegetable purees can thicken sauces. Mashed or pureed potatoes make a good thickener.
- Substitute two egg whites for one whole egg.
- Add vegetables or pastas to meat dishes to decrease the amount of meat (fat) per serving.

Certainly nearly fat-free eating is very possible and very tasty. On the other hand, berries do not quite match the taste sensations of cheesecakes or chocolate mousses. Grilled swordfish may be a real treat, but it does not taste like a porterhouse steak. Unfortunately, high-fat food choices must become "alien food" to you if you expect to lose weight and keep it off forever. You *can* do it. Many, many thousands of people have made the switch to very low-fat eating. It becomes a way of life, and can be very satisfying. In any case, it beats the alternative for those of us who have lost weight. You cannot get to a lower weight and stay there without adopting a very low-fat eating plan.

The following "fat facts," some of which have been reviewed in this chapter, underscore my emphasis on mastering this aspect of eating in order to lose weight and keep it off. Please review them carefully. If you know your enemy well (fat, in this case), then you can defeat it more readily.

- Your body uses very little energy to digest and store high-fat foods (for example, three calories of energy expended to digest 100 calories of bacon); your body uses much more energy to digest carbohydrates (twenty-three calories expended to digest 100 calories of pasta).
- When you eat high-fat foods, the fat goes into storage very quickly—into your billions of hungry extra fat cells. When a never-overweight person eats high-fat foods, the fat goes into the muscles to be used as fuel.
- High-fat foods can cause an increase in appetite for more high-fat foods.
- Highly successful weight controllers report that their current successes, unlike prior weight losses, became permanent when they learned to eat very little fat.

- Goal for fat intake per day: as low as you can go: aim for 0, accept 20g per day maximum.

The following case provides an excellent example of how one of my clients focused her weight loss efforts on *very* low-fat eating. This focus led to great consistency and very satisfying long-term results.

Connie's Permanent Twenty Pound Weight Loss: "It's my body—that's the way it works."

Connie was sixty-one when we first met three years ago. She owns a successful, but very stressful, small business with twenty-seven employees and is happily married to her second husband, who is in a similar line of work. She lived primarily in Chicago, but spent a lot of time commuting to a distant suburb, where her ex-husband and their two grown daughters lived. She also did considerable traveling for work. In fact, she estimated that she ate approximately one-third her meals at restaurants.

Connie was quite happy in her work and with her second marriage (seven years at the time of our initial meeting). However, she was very dissatisfied with her weight and fitness levels. She had been used to living her life as a trim, five-foot-four, 130-pound woman who was fairly athletic. Over the past ten years, however, as life had become more complex with more commuting and less available time, her exercising became more sporadic and her weight increased by twenty-four pounds. Although she was not substantially overweight and the health risks of this amount of excess weight were modest, it really bothered her a great deal to feel as though she was in a body, as she said, that "wasn't right for me."

Connie's main barriers to successful and permanent weight control were:

- Inconsistent exercise and sedentary living
- Excessive drinking (one to two glasses of wine, sometimes much more, quite often)
- Often minimal eating early in the day or midday, with excessive eating in the evening
- Some variability in consumption of fat (e.g., regular salad dressings on salads; bar food fairly often)

Connie had one perfect tendency for a weight controller: She liked looking at the details of her life. She was not at all adverse to self-monitoring, measuring and focusing on exactly what she ate, how she moved and the circumstances that affected her either positively or negatively. She and I used this tendency to her advantage by encouraging her to use her PDA to keep careful track of her eating and exercising. She did this religiously and enjoyed the process. She also began incorporating a more consistent eating pattern, beginning in the morning and including a modest lunch. She loved and sought out vegetable sandwiches, essentially salads between two slices of bread, usually with mustard as a condiment.

Connie and I did not focus directly on decreasing drinking alcoholic beverages, even though it might be a problem. She didn't want to modify her drinking and believed she could incorporate it at a moderate level into a healthy lifestyle.

The following food records were obtained approximately six months after Connie started her program with me. She had already lost all twenty-two pounds by the time this example of her food record began. So, these records suggest what worked for Connie (and still works for her, five years after beginning this effort). You will note in these records that she ate very limited amounts of fat. She and I both saw that as a critical aspect of her success. What does not appear in these records, but was included in Connie's actual daily records, was her exercising. This included at least thirty minutes of exercise virtually every single day—generally walking, running, using a treadmill, some strength training and various stretching and related exercises.

Take a look at these food records and consider what elements of Connie's approach you might incorporate into your own patterns. For example, you may wish to avoid using your calories for alcohol the way Connie does, but you might follow her example in minimizing your consumption of fat whenever and wherever possible.

SUGAR: HOW SWEET IT IS—AND ISN'T

Happiness is the reward of an active life that is lived with "sweet reason," according to Aristotle. Writer Susan Cohler made it clear why Americans often indulge in the sweet part of sweet reason:

> *In the harsh light of the suburban ice cream parlor, a gangly adolescent creates a masterpiece. Three scoops of sweet delight nestled side by side, enfolded in the arms of a ripe banana. Steaming fudge drapes the ice cream slopes and snakes its way to the depths of the dish. A cloud of whipped cream,*

Monday, January 6 / Weight: 131.0

		Calories	Fat Grams
7:00 A.M.	Coffee	25	0.5
	Banana/Orange Juice Shake	165	1.0
12:00 Noon	Fruit	200	1.0
7:00 P.M.	Rice	200	0.0
	Shrimp	90	1.0
	Salmon	120	5.0
	Pretzels	100	0.0
	Wine	270	0.0
	Milk	90	0.0
	Frozen Yogurt	120	0.0
	Totals	**1,380**	**8.5**

Tuesday, January 7 / Weight: 130.0

7:00 A.M.	Coffee	25	0.5
	Cereal	140	0.0
12:00 Noon	Veggie Sandwich	180	1.5
	Turkey, 1 slice	20	0.5
8:00 P.M.	Veggies	100	2.0
	Mashed sweet potatoes	200	1.0
	Rolls	60	0.5
	Pretzels	100	0.0
	Frozen Yogurt	120	0.0
	Milk	90	0.0
	Totals	**1,035**	**6.0**

Saturday, January 11 / Weight: 131.0

7:00 A.M.	Cereal	140	0.0
	Coffee	25	0.5
12:00 Noon	Veggie Sandwich	180	1.5
8:00 P.M.	Salad with clear rice noodles	100	0.0
	Wine	180	0.0
	Pretzels	100	0.0
	Frozen Yogurt	120	0.0
	Totals	**845**	**2.0**

bejeweled with nuts and one cherry crowns the top. This ice cream treat is a work of edible art, but what it does to [you]… may be worth thinking about.

Sugar clearly permeates our lives. It can provide the foundation to "edible art," and it plays a major part in almost all of our celebrations (especially Valentine's Day, Easter and Christmas). Think about the well-known phrases "Home sweet home" and "How sweet it is!" Think of many of the most common terms of endearment: sugar, sweetheart, sweetie, cookie, honeybunch, sugar plum and sweet pea. I have personally used many of these terms to refer to my three children. Not only do relationships involve sugar metaphors, but so do our sports performances. Have you seen a sports telecast that did *not* include such phrases as "sweet shot?" Sugar is idealized in these phrases. The best thing you could say about a person is that he or she is sweet.

Loving Sugar

What causes this infatuation with sugar? In fact, some biological roots may help explain it. When we are hungry, sugar provides the quickest antidote. In other words, the sugar you eat is very similar chemically to the primary source of energy in your body—glucose. Sugar is white, refined sucrose that is derived from sugarcane and beets. It is actually composed of glucose, in addition to fructose (fruit sugar). These components are readily split apart in the small intestine by the enzyme sucrase.

Several other factors reveal that sugar's appeal has biological roots. First, sweet foods are safe foods. This harkens back to our earlier discussion of hunter-gatherers. Can you think of any examples of wild fruits, berries or vegetables that are sweet and also dangerous to eat? Probably not. If you find something hanging from a tree and it tastes sweet, it is almost certainly safe to eat. On the other hand, sour or bitter fruits or vegetables are much more likely to be poisonous.

Second, when humans or other animals are starving, they consistently show heightened preferences for very sweet foods. This, again, shows the body's orientation to satisfying extreme hunger and food deprivation quickly and effectively with sugar.

A third factor that reveals the biological roots of sugar's appeal is the body's way of increasing the craving for sugar. When we eat carbohydrates, especially sugar, production of insulin increases. Insulin directs glucose into muscles and other organs. When we eat a sugary snack, a candy bar for example, the body reacts to it by producing an excessive amount of insulin. This probably occurs because the body is programmed to eat large amounts of sugar or sweet foods whenever they are available. This made sense for hunter-gatherers. If they found something that tasted sweet, their bodies wanted to encourage them to eat large quantities of it. So when you eat that candy bar, your body is over-prepared to digest it. This over-preparedness includes an excess amount of insulin that clears the blood of most of its energy supply (glucose). This results in a very low level of glucose in the blood. The brain then detects this low level of glucose and causes a substantial increase in hunger. In other words, **when you eat sugary foods, it creates a bio-chemical chain reaction leading to increased hunger.**

The research that supports these assertions includes studies in which rabbits were fed glucose directly into their stomachs. These rabbits then ate more, after receiving a high dose of sugar, than they did under normal conditions, and quite a bit more than rabbits who received only salt water injected into their stomachs. I've already discussed how fat begets fat; now you can see how sugar begets more sugar.

Mark, a dedicated weight controller, tried to eat all the right things. Early on in his participation in my program, I noticed that he ate muesli regularly for breakfast. Muesli, granola and similar cereals have a reputation for being health foods. After all, they are made from whole grains, contain lots of fiber and are sold in health food stores. Unfortunately, they contain lots of sugar. Sometimes the sugar is in the form of honey. But your body can't tell the difference between honey and other sugars. Honey does contain small amounts of such minerals as potassium and calcium, but you would have to eat two hundred tablespoons of honey to meet the body's daily requirement for calcium.

Mark was persuaded that his muesli wasn't great for him. So, he substituted shredded wheat and was amazed that this simple change resulted in much less hunger throughout the day and dramatically decreased cravings for sweets.

Recently, a new member joined the group in which Mark participated. Linda was eating low-fat granola for breakfast regularly. She also was snacking on candy bars later in the morning and sometimes in the afternoon as well. This pattern had contributed to significant weight gain over the past couple of years. Mark and I persuaded Linda to substitute a low-sugar food for her granola. Agreeing that "it's worth a shot," she began eating a bagel and low-fat cream cheese as an alternative to her usual breakfast of granola. She came back from this experiment saying, "The 'Muesli Syndrome' lives! I can't believe what a difference this made. I'm also amazed that it worked immediately. As soon as I started eating bagels instead of granola, I didn't have that gnawing feeling in my stomach anymore at ten o'clock. Wow!"

Energy Boost:
Candy Versus Ten-Minute Walks

Robert Thayer, a California State University psychologist, conducted an important study demonstrating that sugar can also affect your mood. Thayer compared the effects of eating a half ounce candy bar (of any type) with taking a rapid ten-minute walk. After participants took ten-minute walks, their tension-level ratings decreased very quickly and stayed much lower for two subsequent hours compared to before they walked. In contrast, after they ate the candy bar, tension levels increased over a sixty-minute period and stayed high for the subsequent hour as well.

Similar effects occurred for ratings of energy levels. Subjects indicated feeling more energized for thirty minutes after eating the candy bar, but their energy levels fell to much lower levels one to two hours later. In contrast, after subjects took walks, their energy levels increased dramatically during the first thirty minutes and stayed well above their pre-walk states for two hours afterwards. Eating candy can cause a logy or tired feeling because it stimulates the release of a natural tranquilizer in our brains called serotonin.

These findings are very important. They suggest a good alternative to eating sugary snacks in order to feel energized: A ten minute brisk walk can provide a much better energy boost than a candy bar. You won't find commercials encouraging people to take ten minute walks for that "quick energy boost," though you will find plenty of commercials hawking candy bars for that purpose. Now you know the truth about which works better.

Conclusion

Avoid sugary foods, especially for breakfast and snacks. It is most helpful to avoid eating any snacks that contain lots of sugar, such as candy bars, ice cream cones, granola bars, caramel corn and cookies. Some of these foods have tremendous nostalgic appeal, unfortunately, but it's time to create a new tradition for yourself.

It is also very wise to avoid sugary breakfast cereals. Instead, try low-sugar cereals, bagels, fruit, crackers or raw vegetables. Also, try to take a brief walk to feel energized—sugar just makes you tired and hungry. This approach keeps blood glucose levels relatively stable. It also helps avoid some of the other chemical reactions that produce strong cravings for some very high-calorie (and high-fat) foods.

PROTEIN POWER

"Protein" comes from the Greek word *proteios,* which means "of prime importance." According to the authors of an amazing book about nutrition and health, *The China Study,* "Ever since the discovery of this nitrogen-containing chemical in 1839 by the Dutch chemist Gerhard Mulder, protein has loomed as the most sacred of all nutrients." It is still touted as the most important building block of life by most people today.

We only need about fifty grams of protein per day, but many current diets recommend consuming more than twice that amount. Current dietary recommendations (Institute of Medicine) include a level of protein intake ranging from about forty to 120 grams per day. These numbers are based on the current Dietary Reference Intakes (DRIs). That range varies tremendously based on such factors as activity levels and amounts of muscle being maintained. If we consume about 10 percent of our total calories from protein, then virtually all of us will supply our bodies with adequate amounts of protein. In the USA, we consume 50 percent more than that level on average. For many weight controllers who are actively attempting to lose weight, 10 percent of calories from a total intake of 1200–1500 calories per day would equal only 30–40 grams of protein.

In our Wellspring programs, we target seventy grams of protein per day. This level, more than the minimal number of protein grams required for nutritional health, has been associated, at least in our experience, with substantial weight loss without much hunger or many complaints about the food. You may wish to aim for seventy grams of protein a day as a starting point to see how this affects your appetite control and your pattern of weight loss.

Protein can help you control your weight in several ways. These include:

- Stimulating the release of the digestive hormone Cholecystokinin (more commonly known as CCK).

- Increased release of neurotransmitters associated with feelings of satiety and fullness. CCK helps trigger this release.
- Stabilizing your blood glucose levels by slowing digestion. The brain monitors these blood glucose levels to affect appetite when they get too low.
- Certain elements of proteins (specific amino acids) also trigger the release of neurotransmitters in the brain that decrease hunger.

A recent review by psychologist R.J. Stubbs of the effects of protein versus carbohydrates versus fat on appetite led to the following conclusion:

> *The data derived from a number of sources ranging from diet surveys to whole body calorimetry and nutrient infusion studies suggest that in the short-to-medium term, protein is more satiating that carbohydrate which is more satiating than fat (i.e., satiation order: protein > carbohydrates > fat).*

One simple way of thinking about these findings concerns the complexity of protein molecules. Protein molecules are far more complex than carbohydrate and fat molecules. This complexity causes the body to take more time to digest high-protein foods, resulting in a time-release effect on the amount of glucose (sugar) in our blood streams. The specific qualities of protein also trigger the release of chemicals in the brain (neurotransmitters) somewhat similar to anti-depressants. To obtain these effects consistently, it helps to eat protein consistently throughout the day.

Protein exists in a great many foods, but especially rich sources of protein include legumes (seed bearing plants like soybeans, green beans, peas, lentils and kidney beans), egg whites and lean meats (white meats of poultry, fish and seafood). For example, a half cup of legumes and one ounce of lean meat both contain about ten grams of protein.

A Caveat about Animal vs. Plant Protein: Plant Protein is Probably Better for Your Health

In a very important series of studies, nutritionist Colin Campbell from Cornell University and his associates showed that relatively high levels of animal proteins can increase the development of cancerous cells and tumors in mice and rats. Humans and rats apparently have similar needs for protein. Dr. Campbell used strains of rats and mice which were exposed to a high level of a couple of different types of carcinogens (chemicals that reliably produce cancerous tumors over time). He found that providing these animals with diets that contained 20 percent of calories from animal protein caused dramatic increases in both pre-cancerous cells (called "foci") and actual lethal tumors over time. Quite remarkably, diets containing 5 percent animal protein and 20 percent plant protein did not produce these very harmful effects.

Related findings have apparently been obtained for other types of proteins and other types of cancers based on studies by Dr. Campbell's group and other researchers. However, in his wonderful book that summarized these and related findings, *The China Study*, Dr. Campbell provided the following caution when applying these studies to our lives:

> *So much consistency [in the animal studies] was impressive, but one aspect of this research demanded that we remain cautious: all this evidence was gathered in experimental animal studies. Although there are strong arguments that these provocative findings are qualitatively relevant to human health, we cannot know the quantitative relevance. In other words, are these principles regarding animal protein and cancer critically important for all humans in all situations, or are they merely marginally important for a minority of people in fairly unique situations. (p.66)*

Dr. Campbell and his associates ventured far outside their laboratories in Ithaca, New York, to see if their impressive findings about the potential dangers of animal protein might emerge with humans. They conducted a massive nutritional study in China that involved almost one billion people over twenty years. This study also showed that a diet very low in fat, high in fiber and low in animal protein seems clearly associated with very low incidences of heart disease, cancer and other serious afflictions in affluent cultures like ours. However, even the least active groups of Chinese people who were studied are more active than the vast majority of Americans. So, increased activity was also associated with improved health, as we would expect.

The China study's results were consistent with the animal studies, but such survey research doesn't prove that animal protein at modest levels will prove harmful for most people, most of the time. The Wellspring Plan encourages a very low-fat and high-fiber diet, as well as greatly increased activity levels. Further research may show that even in this context, much smaller amounts of animal protein than expected can produce harmful results. The most cautious approach would be to attempt to eliminate as much animal protein (and fat) from your diet as possible. A less stringent approach would be to aim for no more than 30 grams of animal protein per day, which would be less than 10 percent of calories from protein for most weight controllers. The latter level would provide some protection, as shown by another one of Dr. Campbell's findings, that precancerous foci didn't develop at an accelerated level until a 12 percent animal protein diet was consumed by rats.

Following even the least restrictive recommendation (30 g of animal protein per day) will prove quite challenging for many people. You'll find yourself eating a lot of low-fat tofu, Seitan (a wheat protein meat substitute) and legumes and drinking a lot of soy milk in order to maintain not only your appetite but your long-term health. Fortunately, these foods are now widely available in convenient forms, including frozen low-fat soy cheese pizzas and many other products. Sources of animal protein are among the more calorie-dense foods that people following the Wellspring Plan typically consume. This approach will, therefore, also encourage more low-calorie-density eating—an important element of eating to lose weight described in the next section of this chapter.

GETTING A BIGGER BANG FOR YOUR CALORIES: EATING FOODS THAT ARE LOW IN ENERGY DENSITY

If you could eat as much as you want in order to feel satisfied, in which of the following meals would you wind up consuming more total calories?

| Grilled chicken + seasoned white rice + assorted vegetables + one glass of ice water | Soup made from grilled chicken, seasoned white rice, assorted vegetables, water |

A variety of studies suggest that you would eat about 20 percent more of the food when presented in the usual fashion compared to the soup version. The soup version is low in energy density because the soup contains relatively few calories per ounce. You'd have consumed a good deal of the liquid from the soup when eating it. In contrast, the chicken dish with a glass of water on the side would produce higher energy density in part because you wouldn't drink as much water during that meal. In everyday life, foods that are low in energy density are foods that have low amounts of calories per gram or weight or per ounce in volume. These include vegetables, fruits and very low-fat foods. Foods with the greatest energy density would be such things as chocolate, pastries and high-fat meats and cheeses.

Quite a few studies with animals and humans show that by adding more fluid to meals and decreasing the energy density accordingly, people eat considerably less than they do with the same fat levels at higher density presentations. Some of these studies also show that simply removing some high-density foods from a person's diet has little effect on their total consumption. On the other hand, removing all sources of high-fat foods almost always results in much less eating and much less fat.

Eating low-density foods increases the size of the stomach and that creates a feeling of fullness. Eating such foods also slows down the rate of transfer of nutrients into the small intestines, another mechanism that decreases appetite and increases feelings of fullness.

A study of nearly 1,800 participants conducted in Philadelphia nicely illustrates this point. Greater consumption of soup was associated with better weight loss. Eating soup is a particularly good way of decreasing energy density levels in your diet. Perhaps similar findings would occur if the researchers measured consumptions of salads per week or eating large portions of vegetables every day.

The take-away message from research on energy density is that you will find weight control easier if you focus on low-density foods. In particular, try to eat as much soup as you can and order lots of vegetables when dining out. This will make you feel more satisfied more often, as well as decrease your desire to eat higher-fat foods.

ROUGHING IT: FIBER

Fiber, sometimes called roughage, can cause gas, bloating and other unpleasant side effects (think baked beans). These occasional unpleasant moments bely the fact that fiber can decrease appetite, improve weight loss and reduce the risk of heart disease and some cancers.

According to the Food and Drug Administration, fiber is a nutrient composed of non-digestible carbohydrates. More specifically:

- Dietary fiber consists of non-digestible carbohydrates that are intrinsic and intact in plants.
- Added fiber consists of isolated, non-digestible carbohydrates which have beneficial physiological effects in humans.
- Total fiber is the sum of dietary and added fiber.

Fiber and Weight

Populations that consume lots of fiber have relatively few overweight people. In Kenya, Uganda and Malawi, for example, where less than 15 percent of adults are overweight, people eat more than four times the fiber that we do (60-80 g/day vs. 15 g/day). Could it be mere coincidence that we eat a quarter of the fiber but have more than four times the percentage of overweight people than these high-fiber countries? Here's another statistic worth pondering: even within each country, those who consume more fiber weigh less than those who consume very little fiber.

An important study published in 1995 by Alfieri and her associates compared the effects of providing a fiber supplement versus a placebo supplement to overweight participants. The participants who got the fiber lost significantly more weight and reported significantly less hunger than the placebo group. Fiber supplementation has also improved the maintenance of weight loss in other research.

How Fiber Helps

Fiber acts to reduce the energy density of foods consumed. That makes sense because adding lots of high-fiber vegetables to a meal increases the bulk and weight of the food, without influencing the amount of calories consumed much at all. Consider the example of adding lettuce, tomatoes and bean sprouts to a sandwich—and changing the bread from white to whole grain. These veggies might add thirty calories and the change in bread would add no additional calories, but those changes would add about six grams of fiber (20 percent of the day's goal for fiber).

High-fiber foods also increase chewing, promoting increased production of saliva and stomach acids. Those fluids and the bulk of the food can increase distention of the stomach and decrease the speed of absorption in the intestines. These effects increase feelings of satiation (satisfaction of appetite during eating) and satiety (fullness): satiation + satiety = decreased eating.

Recommendation: 30g+ of Fiber per Day

Health and nutrition experts recommend that we double our current intake of fiber, from fifteen to thirty grams per day. As a weight controller, you need all the help you can get to fight your resistant biology, and the excess hunger this unfortunate biology awakens in you every day. Eating lots of fiber can get your diet lower in energy density and higher in satisfaction. So, consider using some of the following foods regularly to get to a minimum of thirty grams of fiber every day:

- High-fiber breakfast cereals
- Whole grain breads for sandwiches (2 slices = 4g)
- Bean soups or ¼ cup of baked beans or ½ cup of peas, lentils or corn (all = 5g)
- 1 medium white potato with skin or 1 cup of brown rice or ½ cup of whole-grain pasta (all = 4g)
- 3-4 servings of veggies or salad (6 g)
- fresh fruit (1 serving = 3g)

In addition to these suggestions, just consider some side-by-side comparisons and decide which would work best for you:

- Whole-grain Bread (1 slice): **2 g fiber**, 75 calories, 1 fat g, vs. White Bread (same calories and fat): **.7 g fiber**
- Brown Rice (1 cup cooked): 220 calories, 1.5 fat g, **3.2 g fiber** vs. White Rice (1 cup, cooked): 240 calories, .5 fat g, **1.6 g fiber**
- Oranges (2 medium): 140 calories, 0 fat, **7.6 g fiber** vs. Orange Juice (1 12 oz glass): 170 calories, 0 fat, **.5g fiber**.

The first two side-by-side comparisons suggest the strong benefit of adding color to your grain selections whenever possible. This even works for potatoes, with sweet potatoes having 50 percent more fiber than white ones. The last comparison indicates that, as famed nutritionist Allan Borushek, the "Calorie King" (see **www.calorieking.com**), pointed out, when you eat fresh fruit compared to drinking juice, you get high fiber, low calorie density, considerable time chewing, better satisfaction (reduced hunger), slower absorption and less release of insulin. Now, that is a nutritional deal few weight controllers can pass up.

Conclusion about Fiber

To reach a 30+ gram fiber goal every day, you will find yourself ordering double portions of vegetables at restaurants, munching carrots regularly, insisting on whole grain bread for your sandwiches, seeking out whole fruits for snacks and making or ordering soups very often. The more you embrace these routines and make them significant parts of your weight loss program, the better your chances for lifelong success.

EAT YOUR CALORIES—DON'T DRINK THEM

In the previous section, you read about the substantial benefits of eating fresh oranges versus drinking orange juice. The following recent research findings show the problems caused by drinking calorie-laden sweet drinks (including sodas, sports drinks and fruit juices):

- Researchers from Denmark provided overweight volunteers with either sugared soda or diet sodas. The volunteers ate freely otherwise over the ten-week study. Those who drank sugared sodas consumed an extra 500-700 calories a day and gained three and a half pounds. They also increased their blood pressures. Those who drank diet sodas lost two pounds.
- In a study conducted at Purdue University, volunteers were assessed during a baseline period to determine how many calories they typically consumed. Then, during two four-week experimental periods, they were given 18 percent of their baseline calories as either jelly beans (solid sugar calories) or sugared soda (liquid calories). When the volunteers ate the jelly beans, they compensated for the calories in the jelly beans by eating less during the day. In this way, the jelly beans had no effect on their total consumption of calories compared to their baseline eating. In contrast, when they consumed the sugared sodas, they ate more total calories and gained weight.
- David Ludwig and associates at Harvard University found that for each additional sugared drink (juice, soda, sports

drink) consumed by middle-school children, compared to the average middle-schooler, there was a 60 percent increased risk for the development of obesity—even after controlling for the influence of lifestyle and diet.

Even though sugared drinks contain no fat, they clearly create problems for weight controllers. Even the American Pediatric Association now recommends diet sodas over fruit juices for this reason. Fruit juice, even 100 percent fruit juice, provides almost no fiber and lots of concentrated sugary calories that apparently increase the total calories consumed per day.

The major exception to this dictum (eat your calories—don't drink them) involves skim milk. Skim milk contains a good amount of protein (9 grams per glass) and lots of calcium. So, the bottom line is:

Eat Your Calories—Don't Drink Them (Except for Skim Milk).

Drinking occasional light beer and wine also won't destroy your weight control program. These drinks may be important to you in order for you to find foods (and some drinks) you love that love you back. See the next section for more on this key point. On the other hand, if you drink alcohol frequently or excessively on occasion, that could certainly affect your success. Focus drifts from consistent low-fat eating and self-monitoring when filtered by an alcohol-induced high. When people get distracted and less focused in such settings, suddenly chips, nuts and fried chicken wings seem okay. Also, alcoholic drinks contain plenty of calories, especially the kinds that come in colors with small paper umbrellas in them.

CALORIE CONSCIOUSNESS

If you ate unlimited quantities of very low-fat, high-plant-protein, low-density, low-sugar, high-fiber foods, then you would certainly gain a substantial amount of weight. These six elements of eating to lose weight can control your appetite and regulate your weight; however, you have to watch what happens on the scale as you implement this. If your activity levels have increased substantially and you are following these food guidelines but your weight doesn't change, then you have to consider focusing more specifically on the amount of calories you are consuming every day.

The highly successful weight controllers in the National Weight Control Registry studies have lost more than fifty pounds and maintained that weight loss for an average of six years. Their reported average intake per day is approximately 1,350 calories. Based on prior research that verifies reports of eating, it seems likely that this number is a bit low. Let's assume that their average intake is closer to 1,500 or 1,600 calories per day as a maintenance level. **These numbers suggest that a good target for weight loss for most people might be 1,200–1,300 calories per day, in addition to considerable activity.** If you are able to lose weight consistently simply by following the other six elements in this chapter and increasing your activity levels, then focusing very specifically on the calories consumed will not help you. However, to accelerate weight loss or to begin weight loss for some people, these levels of caloric consumption can guide your eating. In addition, many of my clients find that one other caloric guideline has proven particularly helpful:

Consume no more than 800 calories at your biggest meal of the day.

This useful goal can help you when you're grappling with a menu at an Italian restaurant, for example. Many restaurants serve enormous portions of pasta that by themselves can greatly exceed 800 calories.

A recent report from the Centers for Disease Control shows why some attention to calorie consumption matters. According to this report, over the last thirty years men have eaten 168 more calories daily than they did in 1971. They now eat, according to self-reports, approximately 2,600 calories a day. Women have consumed 335 more calories over these past thirty years, increasing their total calorie consumption to approximately 1,900 calories per day. Most nutritionists would argue that most people actually consume even more than these self-reports suggest. For example, Susan Roberts of the Energy Metabolism Lab at Tufts University noted that more than six in ten Americans are either overweight or obese. She points out that we didn't get there on 1,900 to 2,600 calories per day and that U.S. food supply data indicates that Americans are eating considerably more than they used to.

This means that if you are a serious weight controller, then you'll consume about half of what average Americans consume per day. You'll also expend far more energy than typical Americans, eat less fat and eat more fiber and more low-density food. When you deviate so much from the average tendencies of those around you, you must rely on a good deal of inner strength to stay the course.

FIND LOVABLE FOODS THAT LOVE YOU BACK

The thing I love about a good steak is its hardiness; its stick-to-your-ribs quality. It just looks and smells like it's going to feel so good going down. I like it burned around the edges, pinkish in the middle, sizzling hot. I know I'll feel satisfied and nicely full and relaxed after a good steak. Steaks may cost some serious bucks, but they're a lot cheaper than [depressants].

*A couple of scoops of really rich chocolate or vanilla fudge ice cream just call out to me sometimes. I just love the smooth, creamy texture and the taste sensation of rich ice cream. It creates this ahhhhhhhhhhhh and yummmmmmmmmmm feeling that is both exciting and relaxing simultaneously. What else in life does that? Well, I guess I can think of something—but you can't buy **that** 24 hours a day at your nearest convenience store, or maybe you can but I just don't know how.*

*Nothing smells as good as freshly baked chocolate chip cookies! I mean **nothing**. When they just come out of the oven, piping hot, they really take over the room. They bring me back to a simpler time, with my brother and sister laughing and excitedly arguing about who gets the first one. That melt-in-your-mouth warmth and sweetness is just one of the great parts of being human.*

What makes your favorite foods lovable? Lovable foods have certain qualities in common:

- Look really good
- Smell great
- Taste great
- Have mouth appeal—chewy or crunchy or just right for the moment
- Create good, happy and satisfied feelings
- Are craved for their special qualities

- Have some nostalgic value, reminders of something good from the past, like warm family gatherings or very relaxing or romantic moments
- Provide comfort, relief from stress

Such qualities abound in juicy steaks, rich ice creams and freshly baked cookies. I have heard friends describe, in amazing detail, the lovable qualities of freshly baked lemon meringue pies, rich beers and perfect pizzas. We talk about such foods with a certain reverence, elevating them to romantic heights.

Weight Controllers Can Keep Their Passions for Food and Still Succeed

Passion makes life more interesting. Living the good life includes enjoying good food passionately. If you minimize your interest in food, making food bland and unappealing, you can expect to fail in the quest for permanent change. Among the thousands of clients I have worked with over the past forty years, those who have achieved long-term success have kept the passion in their food and in other parts of their lives. In short, by cherishing your passion for food, you can help yourself lose weight permanently.

Four Aspects of Lovable Foods

If you learn the details about the lovability of food, you might be able to increase your enjoyment of it and your passion for it. Identifying these qualities is just the beginning of understanding how passion for food really works.

Consider your reaction if you went to a fancy, expensive restaurant and all the food was presented wrapped in layers of paper, like a fast-food meal. Would that presentation affect your reaction to the food? What if you ordered chicken soup on a cold wintry day and it came out cold and clammy? Would a frozen yogurt cone appeal to you as much if it were served warm and drippy?

Obviously, lovability in foods goes far beyond mere taste sensations. Restaurants go to great pains to set the stage for their food. They know that presentation affects lovability in their foods and they want you to love their food and come back for more, again and again. To assist you in your quest to find lovable foods that love you back, let's consider all the factors that affect the appeal of food. **By increasing your awareness of each factor, you can get more lovability out of your food.**

Table 7-2 describes the four factors. Taste, the most obvious one, consists of various combinations of sweet, sour, salty and bitter. Consider the simple pretzel, for example. If you eat a pretzel in a quiet, dark room and eat it slowly and attentively you'll certainly notice the saltiness, but you'll also detect sweetness. You might even find that the inside of the pretzel, the dry white stuff, tastes a little bitter, at least compared to the outside's salty-sweet shell.

**Table 7-2
Four Lovability Factors**

Taste	*Smell*
• sweet	• pleasing, appropriate for type of food
• salty	• displeasing, foul, inappropriate
• sour	
• bitter	• strong vs. weak
Appearance	*Texture*
• attractive, beautiful	• creamy
• unattractive, ugly	• crunchy
• pleasing setting	• chalky
• fresh	• smooth
• stale, spoiled	• chewy

What happens if you pay attention to each aspect of taste? My clients say they appreciate and enjoy their food more when they get themselves to do this. The quick, salty pretzel snack becomes something that is a little sweet, quite salty, a little bitter and a bit more interesting and enjoyable.

Now what happens if you put the pretzels on a hand-crafted oak platter, next to several porcelain cups with various mustards in them, on top of a glistening round antique oak table? Wouldn't their appeal increase compared to the appeal of a plastic bag of pretzels being munched in your car? Appearance definitely matters. Smell and texture in food also matter. If your pretzels were stale, rubbery or smelled funny, you'd find them less lovable. If you like coffee, you know that a strong coffee smell and an appealing mug and setting in which to drink it all affect its lovability.

You can use all four aspects of the lovability of food to make your low-fat world much more enjoyable. Consider trying the following lovability enhancers as often as possible:

- **Accentuate taste** by eating slowly and attempting to identify the degree to which whatever you eat tastes sweet, salty, sour and bitter. You can think of this as savoring your food by making yourself aware of each element of its taste.
- **Maximize the appearance** of food that you serve yourself. This applies even when eating your food out of a microwavable box. It helps to put the food on a nice plate and sit down at a pleasant table for your meal. You can try adding candles, place settings and flowers to create your own beautiful ambiance.
- **Enjoy the smells** of food. All food smells are fat-free and calorie free! You can try this at coffee shops, cheese counters and other places where strong appealing smells waft through the air. For your own food, take time to identify the smells and notice what you enjoy about each of them.
- **Pay attention to texture** in everything you eat. You can enjoy luxurious textures in very low-fat foods quite readily. Can you think of chewy fat-free foods that you sometimes enjoy (hint: gum, turkey jerky)? Certainly frozen yogurts can vary in creaminess, and lots of healthful snacks have plenty of crunch, like carrots, pretzels and most fresh vegetables. For smooth qualities, smoothies and even certain cereals can prove satisfying.

Sweet Potatoes:
A Lovable Food that Loves You Back

Lovable foods can certainly, definitely and without a doubt include foods that *love you back*. Foods that help you lose weight, achieve your goals, make you healthier, that are constructive rather than destructive, can fulfill all of the qualities of traditional lovable foods.

The same clients who waxed poetic about steaks and chocolate sundaes have talked lovingly about sweet potatoes:

- "Sweet potatoes are treats: colorful, easy, tasty."
- "They fill me up—and do it with warmth and flavor."
- "They remind me of holidays, obviously Thanksgiving, but also Christmas. I remember the sweet smell of them, bubbling out of the oven with marshmallows on top; definite yums for yams from my family."
- "They're interesting; you can do so much with them—making them crunchy or soupy or topping them with a whole world of possibilities. Usually I top them with a honey mustard, for a sweet and tangy taste, but they also work really well with different fruit salsas or barbecue sauces or yogurts."
- "I know that when I get home, I'm nine minutes away from something sweet, filling and satisfying."

My clients talk about remembering celebrating Thanksgivings and the comfort and warmth of family. Certainly not all of their families were warm and comfortable, nor was the Thanksgiving holiday always a wonderful, satisfying experience. Yet positive memories for most of us include the smells of turkey and sweet potatoes filling a household on a cold, brisk afternoon, intermingling with a crackling wood fire and the sounds of a football game echoing from a nearby television set.

Sweet potatoes have their place as warm, comfortable, celebratory food in many of our hearts and minds. Can you see a sweet potato casserole in your memory and remember the oohs and aahs from the family gathered together? Can you remember the feeling of warm excitement that you felt as a child when the food first came out of the oven? Lovable foods can bring these associations back to life.

As with all lovable foods, you can eat sweet potatoes with gusto. One of my clients, Casey, said she could keep losing weight "as long as the sweet potato farmers stay in business." She likes their convenience, warmth, taste, amazing filling quality, variations (with different toppings, for example) and smell. Casey's story, below, highlights her sheer enjoyment of food, eaten now as a successful weight controller.

Casey: "Just Keep Growing Those Sweet Potatoes, PLEASE!"

Casey described her struggle with weight control as something that was always with her. She was preoccupied by "my fat, my pathetic eating." At forty years old and 5'6", she weighed 242 pounds when she first came to my office. Many areas of her life seemed to be fine. She had a new job that she loved, children who were in college and doing well. She was divorced (twice) but had a man in her life whom she loved and felt loved by. Even her finances were beginning to improve. Her new job, after eight months of unemployment, was helping a lot. She saw opportunities and causes for excitement and satisfaction in almost all aspects of her life.

But her eating and her weight just seemed hopeless. Every day she felt annoyed and disappointed in herself: "My kids love and trust me. I've got this great new job, full of challenges and prospects. Barry, my love, is wonderful. How can I keep myself so miserable by eating like I do?" Her cholesterol was too high and her blood pressure was borderline. She took medications to regulate these problems but felt dependent on them. The twinges in her back and other aches and pains made her feel old before her time. She also hated the way she looked. She tried to make some outfit work every day before leaving the house, knowing that everything was just a bit too tight or just didn't look right on her body.

The very first week she started my program she made an immediate transformation to very low-fat eating, daily exercising, extended walks both to and from her car and during the lunch hour and careful journaling of her eating and exercising. By far the most dramatic change in her life was the discovery that she could love to eat foods that could love her back. She began having sweet potatoes every day for dinner, really big ones that she dressed up in various ways. She was shocked by how much she could enjoy really healthy eating. Enjoyment was the key. She found ways of loving foods that were constructive, not destructive. Although her job involved going to restaurants, she learned to make every type of restaurant work for her. Over and over again, as her weight decreased by one to two pounds per week, she was surprised and pleased by how wonderful it felt to finally be getting her problem under control.

After one year and having lost fifty-seven pounds, Casey still expresses wonderment about the quality of her food and the amazing transformations in her life. She loves her new clothes and the sense of strength that she has enjoyed by increasing her exercising and her everyday activities. On many occasions she has talked about not being able to imagine ever going back to eating foods with even modest amounts of fat in them. She says, "Why should I eat other things? I really love this stuff. If you look for it, it's all around you, and it's just wonderful!" Casey has learned that weight control can work without deprivation. It requires passion for food, comfort in food and appreciation of foods that can love you back.

A Nutritional Champ

As you have seen, sweet potatoes are one of the foods that can love you back. Every survey of nutritional qualities of foods puts sweet potatoes at or near the top of the food chain. For example, the consumer watchdog group Center for Science in the Public Interest (CSPI) has scored qualities of foods over the years by adding up their percentages of recommended values for various vitamins, minerals, cancer-fighting elements and fiber. In at least two of these ratings, sweet potatoes outscored every other food by a wide margin. In one of the surveys, a medium baked sweet potato scored 184; the next highest score was 83, awarded to a medium baked regular potato. Another survey using a different scoring system put sweet potatoes on top again (582 points), 148 points above carrots, the second place finisher (434 points).

Table 7-3 shows the nutrients in sweet potatoes compared with white potatoes. As you can see, both types of potatoes are very good foods. For example, both are almost fat-free, cholesterol free and very low in salt (sodium). But the sweet potato stands out for several of its nutritional aspects:

- Medium baked sweet potatoes have 19.3 percent fewer calories than medium baked white potatoes.
- Sweet potatoes have 50 percent more dietary fiber, a major aid in digestion and a means of providing fullness and assisting in hunger control. If a white potato is eaten with skin, however, that can more than double its fiber content. Few people eat sweet potato skins (too bitter).
- Sweet potatoes have more than three times the minimal level of beta carotene (supplying three times more Vitamin A) than white potatoes. It would take twelve cups of broccoli to provide the same amount.
- A medium sweet potato provides three times more Vitamin E than a medium baked potato. Most foods that are rich in Vitamin E (such as vegetable oils, nuts and avocados) also contain lots of fat. This makes sweet potatoes a nutritional bargain for Vitamin E because they have virtually no fat.
- A medium sweet potato provides at least 10 percent of the recommended levels of potassium, manganese, selenium and zinc.

These astounding nutritional qualities make it clear why dietitians place sweet potatoes near the top of virtually all of their lists of "superfoods." Just the Vitamin A content of sweet potatoes makes them truly extraordinary, as it is helpful for healthy eyes, skin, mucus

Table 7-3
Nutrients in Potatoes

	Sweet Potato: medium, baked (2" diameter x 5" long, 114 g)	White Potato: medium, baked (2 1/3" diameter x 4 3/4" long, 156 g)
Calories (kcal)	117	145
Carbohydrate (g)	28	34
Protein (g)	2	3
Fat (g)	0.1	0.2
Dietary Fiber (g)	3.4	2 (eaten with skin: 4.8 g fiber)
Calcium (mg)	32	8
Iron (mg)	0.5	0.6
Magnesium (mg)	23	39
Manganese (mg)	0.6	0.3
Phosphorus (mg)	63	78
Potassium (mg)	397	610
Sodium (mg)	11	8
Selenium (mg)	0.8	0.5
Zinc (mg)	0.3	0.5
Copper (mg)	0.2	0.3
Vitamin A IU	24877	0
Vitamin C (mg)	28	20
Vitamin E (mg)	0.3	0.1
Thiamin (mg)	0.1	0.2
Riboflavin (mg)	0.1	.03
Folate (mcg)	26	14
Niacin (mg)	0.7	2.2
Pantothenic acid (mg)	0.7	.09

membranes, bone growth, tooth development, embryonic growth and immunity mechanisms for fighting infection and disease. Vitamin A may even help the body regulate its time clock. Deficiencies in Vitamin A can cause night blindness, problems with the production of tears and heightened vulnerability to a variety of conditions leading to complete loss of vision. Although these eye diseases are rare in the well-nourished United States, up to 500,000 children a year lose their sight because of deficiencies in Vitamin A. Perhaps most exciting in recent years has been research showing that the building blocks for Vitamin A that come from plants (the carotenoids) may prevent several kinds of cancer, including lung, stomach, larynx, esophageal, bladder, colon, rectal and prostate cancer. Sweet potatoes provide a remarkable amount of beta-carotene, one of the three types of carotenoid building blocks for Vitamin A (alpha-carotene and beta-cryptoxanthin are the others).

History and Variety of Sweet Potatoes

When you realize the extraordinary nutritional qualities of sweet potatoes, you can appreciate that one of Christopher Columbus's greatest unheralded discoveries may have been the sweet potato, which he introduced to Europe in the late 1400s using a Native American name, written in several ways: "batatas," "patate" and "potat." Europeans then referred to sweet potatoes as "potatoes" until the white potatoes we know landed there and were also called "potato." To create a distinction, the orange-fleshed vegetable originally called "potato" in Europe was renamed "sweet potato."

The distinction becomes more complicated when you realize that not only do sweet potatoes differ in many ways from potatoes, but they also differ dramatically from what we call "yams." The sweet potato is a member of the plant family known as the "morning glory," a prehistoric vegetable that serves as a root to store fluids and food for a larger plant. The most common varieties in the United States are moist, sweet and bright orange in color. In contrast, both white potatoes and yams are "tubers," which are stems, not roots, and are dry, starchy and generally white or pale yellow in color.

The confusion of true yams (pale tubers) with sweet potatoes (orange storage roots) started in the 1930s when promoters of Southern-grown sweet potatoes began using the term "yam" to distinguish theirs from the drier, paler sweets grown in Northern climates (New Jersey, Maryland and Virginia). To this day, many grocery stores mislabel one or more variations of actual sweet potatoes as yams. To avoid confusion, just remember that true yams are paler in color than most sweet potatoes, rarely sweet, derived from a different part of the plant and are generally not readily available in the United States.

There are three types of sweet potatoes considered traditional in North American markets: Beauregard, Jewel and Garnet. These orange-fleshed types have a moist and decidedly sweet quality when cooked. Most of the other sweet potatoes that are sometimes available here are lighter toned, even white in color, and much drier and less sweet in taste than the traditional orange varieties. The most common non-orange types are the Boniato and Asian sweet potatoes. "Asian" in this regard is a market catchall term for various rose-skinned, ivory-flesh versions developed in the East. When baked, these sweet potatoes turn yellow with a smooth and medium-dry texture. The traditional orange types are clearly sweeter, much more moist, have greater nutritional value (particularly Vitamin A) and are strongly preferred by most Americans.

Mike's Dilemma: Sweet Potato vs. Bagel

My client Mike overcame his overeating (over-grazing) by transforming his passion for a classic dieter's food that can pile on pounds if overeaten into a passion for sweet potatoes. When I first met Mike, almost two years ago, he was not the kind of person who sat down to one or two big meals a day, but was a classic grazer. He preferred a bit here, a nibble there, a snack here and a munch there. This style of eating has many advantages, believe it or not. More frequent meals create more frequent demands on your body, which has to work harder to digest food when it's consumed more often. This in turn raises your metabolic rate, the rate at which your body burns energy just to keep you alive and breathing. That can help you lose weight without requiring you to exercise more or eat less.

But one of Mike's challenges was that he often grazed on foods that were high in calories, sometimes surprisingly so. For example, he often ate several bagels per day. Bagels used to be relatively small, very chewy and clearly a very low-fat, tasty food. But, in recent years they have grown, with some topping the scale at several ounces, therefore several hundred—sometimes 400-500—calories. Mike discovered that sweet potatoes have many advantages over bagels:

Two Days in Mike's Life

Day/Date:	Thursday, 2/28		
Exercise:	35 Min. Treadmill		
Steps:	10,600		
Time	Food	Calories	Fat Grams
7:00 A.M.	Skim Milk	80	0.0
	2 Slices Wheat Toast	220	0.0
	Jam	30	0.0
	Lite PB	75	4.0
8:30 A.M.	Coffee, half and half	30	3.0
11:00 A.M.	Hot Chocolate	180	1.0
12:30 P.M.	Chicken Noodle Soup	100	1.0
	Crackers	40	0.0
	Veggie Pizza	200	3.0
	Non-fat Yogurt	200	0.0
4:00 P.M.	Skim Caramel Macchiato	240	1.0
5:00 P.M.	Beef Jerky	70	1.0
7:00 P.M.	Boca Burger	90	1.5
	Sweet potato with	180	0.0
	Non-fat Cheese	40	0.0
	Pasta/Baked Beans	190	0.0
	Totals	**1,965**	**15.5**

Day/Date:	Friday, 3/1		
Exercise:	30 Min. Walk		
Steps:	12,255		
Time	Food	Calories	Fat Grams
7:00 A.M.	Coffee, non-fat half and half	40	0.0
8:30 A.M.	Non-fat iced Frappuccino	300	0.0
10:30 A.M.	Coffee, half and half	30	3.0
Noon	Black-Eyed Pea Soup	200	0.0
	Crackers	100	3.0
3:00 P.M.	Beef Jerky	70	1.0
	Skim Milk	120	0.0
5:00 P.M.	Sweet potato, BBQ Sauce	200	0.0
6:30 P.M.	Low-fat frozen dinner	240	2.5

	Artichoke with Ground Turkey Breast	160	1.5
	Parmesan Cheese	30	1.5
	Skim Milk	80	0.0
8:00 P.M.	Coffee/Hot Chocolate	170	3.0
10:00 P.M.	Non-fat Frozen Yogurt	200	0.0
	Totals	**1,940**	**15.5**

Mike added, "I work in a mall that has a diverse food court. It includes a great bagel place, but also a grill that bakes potatoes and sweet potatoes. I found the warmth and variety of sweet potatoes makes them far more filling with far fewer calories. (I make it interesting by adding different sauces, like mustards and barbecue sauces.) I've noticed that if I eat a good-sized sweet potato, my interest in food is gone for quite a few hours. For someone like me, who loves to graze, this is a huge benefit."

Mike, with the help of his very supportive wife, Sheila, found that following the principles in this book allowed them both to lose substantial amounts of weight. Mike has lost forty of the fifty pounds he wanted to lose and his wife lost her total goal of twenty pounds. They've succeeded in maintaining these losses and have found that the substitutions they've made, like the sweet potatoes for bagels, have left them enjoying their food more than they did before they went on my weight-loss program. They now enjoy not only the experience of eating, but also the satisfying feeling of eating constructively, not destructively. That sense of accomplishment feels far better than guilt and self-blame.

I've also had clients who developed passions for low-fat soups or cheeseless pizzas. One young client, Rob, began his march to success as a clearly chubby ten-year-old who was four and a half feet tall and weighed 155 lbs. One of Rob's food groups became cheese-less pizza. He either pulled the cheese off his pizza or ordered pizza made without the cheese. At least three times a week (sometimes three times a day!), Rob wrote "pizza, no cheese" in his daily eating journal. Eleven years later, Rob now stands more than a foot taller (5'11") and weighs nearly the same (165 lbs.). If you could grow a foot, you too might find your current weight far more acceptable. Unfortunately, almost all seriously overweight pre-teens become obese adults. Rob learned to find foods that he loved that loved him back and thus avoided the usual pathway from obese pre-teenager to obese adult.

Cheese-less pizza may not work for you as a primary food as it did for Rob. Perhaps sweet potatoes will become a mainstay for you or broth-based Asian stir-fries or buffalo burgers or turkey hot dogs and beans or some other concoction. The recipes in the final chapter may give you other ideas for lovable foods that love you back. You just have to keep experimenting until you find those lovable foods that bring you comfort, joy and interest and keep you healthy. The Wellspring Plan works with pleasurable, healthy foods, not with diets and deprivation.

EXCEPTIONS?

Question: *What about pizza? Pizza, after all, has all the food groups.*

Pizzas often contain vegetables, dairy, meat and grains. They do, indeed, provide a wide range of food groups. This fact would be very important if you were starving on a desert island. However, pizza also contains many calories and many of those calories come from fat. For example, two slices of a national fast food pizza chain's stuffed pizza contains 860 calories and forty grams of fat (42 percent of the calories come from fat). Even this pizza chain's less caloric pizzas, as well as the largest national chain's full range of pizza offerings, contain 30 to 50 percent of the calories from fat. That's three to five times more than your goal in this program. Pizza cheese (mozzarella), made with part-skim milk, is *still* a high-fat food and pizzas often have a lot of cheese on them.

The good news is that many places will serve pizzas without any cheese, which does represent a good food choice. The crust in most pizzas contains some fat (usually one to two grams per slice), but as an alternative food, pizzas with no cheese can work very well.

If you are trapped in a party or meeting and surrounded by pizzas, what can you do? You can remove the cheese from your pizza. Some people may find this distasteful and although not the most acceptable form of behavior, it could work a lot better for you than eating high-fat food.

Question: *What about frozen yogurt?*

Most frozen yogurts are enjoyable low-fat desserts. However, some of them can be surprisingly high in fat content and, therefore, deviate from the plan. If you are selective and read labels carefully, you can find low-fat or no-fat frozen yogurts. But remember that most frozen yogurts contain lots of sugar or other sweeteners and this could trigger some of the same reactions that other sugary foods do.

Many weight controllers use frozen yogurt in modest amounts as a treat, which is a good approach. Just be careful of some establishments that serve nearly twice the amounts that they advertise for a given price. Try ordering the smallest, child-size portion available at a frozen yogurt stand or restaurant. Frozen yogurt can also become problematic if it is purchased in pints, quarts or larger bulk quantities. Many people find themselves dipping into these treats more often than desirable. So the answer is—use frozen yogurt with caution. Frozen yogurt popsicles help many weight controllers control portion sizes when enjoying this treat.

Question: *What about birthday cake?*

Birthday cakes are an important tradition to many people. However, traditions can change. Why would you want to eat a food that creates a problem for you in celebration of a special day? When you first had a cake to celebrate your birthday during childhood, you didn't realize the kind of problem that foods high in sugar and fat create for you. In fact, at that time, you probably didn't have such a problem. Now, you have new information that advises against consuming foods like cake. In the 1950s, practically every dinner table had red meat on it, but that tradition has changed. It is now time for you to consider changing the birthday cake tradition for yourself. This position may seem rather extreme, but weight control takes extreme focusing and persistence. If you really want to succeed at this difficult challenge, you must take difficult steps.

Another problem with allowing yourself birthday cake is that if you give yourself permission for this deviation from the plan, what else will you permit? What about other holidays? What about other people's birthdays? What about your children's birthdays? Some of the clients with whom I have worked give themselves permission to eat problematic foods when they are hungry, tired, on vacation, at someone else's house or are sad or depressed. The list goes on and on.

Permissions often create problems. For example, if you give yourself permission to eat problematic food today, then you may struggle mightily with other food decisions tomorrow. These struggles take their toll. Instead of food becoming more secondary in your life, the struggle becomes primary. Lots of struggles can put you into a major frustration stage—an unpleasant stage that often produces unfavorable results. Can all of these problems come from a birthday cake? Perhaps!

Question: *How can you tell about sauces in restaurants?*

You can assume that any sauce made in a restaurant with oil as a primary ingredient is problematic. On the other hand, tomato sauces and sauces that are essentially broths (which are available increasingly in restaurants) are quite acceptable. Any sauces made with cheese (such as Alfredo sauce) are very high in fat; similarly, sauces and soups with cream bases are very high-fat foods. One of my clients recently told a story about a seemingly innocuous mushroom soup which her dining companion ordered. Her companion raved about how wonderful the soup was, and it looked very appealing to the client. But when she tasted the soup, she realized that its primary ingredient was butter. The word "mushroom" suggests a low-fat, safe, vegetable base. As people all over the world become increasingly health-conscious, restaurateurs and food packagers will market and name products to suggest their healthfulness. You can generally assume that if you're not sure about the ingredients in a product, it's best to avoid it. In a restaurant, try to order only items for which you know the fat and sugar contents. These guidelines may sound stringent, but unfortunately your biology demands such stringencies. Successful weight controllers follow these guidelines with tremendous consistency.

EATING AND CANCER: CAN YOU PREVENT CANCER BY EATING BETTER?

Cancer strikes ten million people per year. Three to four million of those cancers could have been prevented through healthier eating and exercise. In fact, eating more fruits and vegetables alone could eliminate as many as 2 million new cases of cancer a year.

Recently, the World Cancer Research Fund and the American Institute for Cancer Research issued a comprehensive report on the relationship between eating and cancer. This report, based on a careful review of more than 4,500 studies, stressed that no food or drink can prevent cancer, but concluded that a diet that emphasizes certain foods can certainly lower your risk of getting this deadly disease.

In addition to decreasing consumption of animal protein based on the research described in *The China Study*, five eating and drinking strategies that almost certainly can decrease the risk of getting cancer are:

1. **Eat lots of VEGETABLES.** The average American eats only three or four servings a day of vegetables and fruits. Five servings are clearly preferable and nine are recommended by virtually all nutritional experts. Yellow, dark green and orange vegetables rich in carotenoids, and all the cabbage family vegetables (broccoli, Brussels sprouts, cauliflower, collards, kale, bok choy and mustard/turnip greens) all seem to lower the risk of cancer. Garlic, onions and leeks may also help ward off cancer, especially breast cancer.

2. **Eat Lots of FRUITS.** Fruits that are rich in vitamin C (all citrus fruits, tomatoes and strawberries) are especially helpful.

3. **Decrease consumption of total FAT, particularly saturated fat.** Fats should provide between 15 and 30 percent of total calories. You may recall that I have recommended that you go "as low as you can go" in total fat. For most, this may amount to 10 percent of your total calories in fat or slightly more.

4. **Decrease ALCOHOL consumption; limit drinks to less than two a day for men and one a day for women.** The report concluded that although alcohol may have some benefits for decreasing heart disease when consumed in small amounts, the risk for cancers, particularly breast, colon and rectal cancers, is significant. People who consume even small amounts of alcohol show a significantly greater chance of developing cancer than those who do not drink alcohol at all.

5. **The following other foods and drinks may also help reduce the risk of cancer, at least somewhat: dried beans, milk, fish, green tea, whole-grain cereals and olive oil.** The evidence favoring these particular foods and drinks

is not as convincing as the evidence in the first four recommendations. Nonetheless, the panel concluded that those items may prove beneficial and are worth including in healthy eating plans.

SUMMARY AND CONCLUSIONS

Table 7-4 summarizes the eight key principles of eating and drinking in the Wellspring Plan. It also provides ratings of importance, with the four most important principles appearing bolded for emphasis.

Table 7-4
Eight Keys to Eating to Lose Weight and Their Importance for Weight Controllers

1= minimally important, 10= extremely important

1. **Eat very little fat** (aim for 0g, accept <20g per day). Importance = 10

2. Control your consumption of sugar. Importance = 4

3. Eat lean sources of protein frequently throughout the day, substituting plant for animal sources of protein as much as possible (70g total protein;< 30g from animal sources). Importance = 4

4. **Consume low-density foods** (e.g., lots of soups and vegetables). Importance = 8

5. Eat at least 30g of fiber per day. Importance = 3

6. Eat your calories—don't drink them. Importance = 7

7. **Stay calorie conscious** (e.g., maximum calories for biggest meal of the day = 800). Importance = 9

8. **Find lovable foods that love you back.** Importance = 8

Focusing on consuming as little fat as possible will help you implement the other seven elements. When you eat a very low-fat diet, you will naturally gravitate to low-density foods because fat is by far the most calorically dense nutrient (nine calories per gram versus four calories per gram for protein and carbs). Decreasing fat also leads to eating relatively few animal sources of protein. For example, the vast majority of red meats are very high in fat. Low-density and very low-fat foods also have lots of fiber, and so on. So, start your focus with the goal of near zero fat intake and you'll get to the most healthful diet, full of foods you love that love you back. This approach clearly does not focus on moderation. Moderation simply does not work for weight controllers.

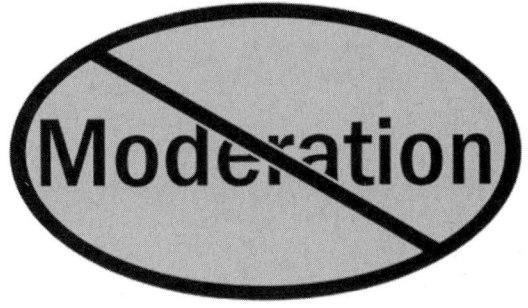

CHAPTER 8

Step 4—Use Movement to Level the Playing Field

Do any of these benefits of movement surprise you? Activity can:

- Increase weight loss
- Improve maintenance of weight loss
- Improve stress management
- Improve quality of sleep
- Improve digestion
- Improve metabolism of fat
- Enhance self-esteem
- Improve resistance to illness
- Increase energy levels
- Reduce blood pressure
- Increase flexibility
- Increase metabolic rate
- Build strength
- Decrease depression
- Increase endorphins (internally produced opiates that improve mood and feelings of well-being)
- Decrease appetite
- Increase lifespan

Most people find this list impressive but still fail to act on it. In fact, the single greatest predictor of long-term success in weight control is activity level. But most adults do not get nearly enough activity to produce many of these health, emotional or hedonic benefits. In fact, only 20 percent of adults over the age of twenty-five engage in physical activity at least twice per week.

Perhaps the most remarkable thing about the benefits of activity is that weight controllers don't have to exercise in the traditional sense in order to get most of these benefits. One of the most useful activities is walking and studies of successful weight controllers reveal that this is the preferred form of activity: the average master of weight control walks briskly for one hour each day.

The best thing about walking is it doesn't require a gym membership or a nearby club or sports team. Let's consider in more detail how you can get yourself to adopt this activity more consistently by taking more steps every day.

KEY GOAL: 12,000+ STEPS A DAY

At Wellspring Camps, most of the teenage participants scoff at 12,000 steps. Wellspring campers average a remarkable 24,000 steps per day. About 2000 steps equals a mile and adults average 4,000 steps per day, but most of that comes from just everyday activities, not from deliberate efforts to get to the goal. So the difference is about 8,000 steps per day. That's about an hour or so of *additional* walking each day and less time if the activity involves moving faster than walking.

BUYING PEDOMETERS

Pedometers are remarkable devices that sit on your hip and count each step you take. Some cheaper pedometers do this with a spring mechanism that may not measure steps accurately. The better pedometers involve a sensitive ball-like mechanism that moves up and down with your stride, as the elevation of your hip changes ever so slightly. More high-tech versions appear now as apps on smart phones and via remarkable devices that you can wear as a bracelet and download information about steps taken, calories burned, time spent in sedentary behaviors and even time of day.

Wearing a pedometer (or related device) can provide you with critical and immediate feedback about your progress relative to the daily goal of 12,000 steps. The pedometer revolution started in Japan about forty years ago and made its way to the US and Canada after researchers at the Cooper Clinic in Dallas demonstrated the device's importance in promoting activity. You can get an accurate pedometer for about twenty dollars.

Rather than purchasing just one pedometer, buy one for every member of your family. If all family members wear a pedometer, pedometers will feel more normal for the weight controllers and increasing your walking will become a common goal. Family members will endorse parking further away from destinations or walking up and down stairs just to get more steps. The research on the use of pedometers demonstrates these effects; just wearing them increases steps and wearing them after setting goals increases steps even more.

THE ADVANTAGES OF FOCUSING ON STEPS

The Wellspring Plan uses the KISSeS principle—Keep It Scientific, Simple and Sustainable. The goal of 12,000 steps also meets all three S's.

- **Scientific:** Successful weight controllers move a lot more than average people. In general, maintaining a high level of activity helps maintain weight loss more than any other single factor that has been studied. For example, Ross Andersen and his colleagues from Johns Hopkins University School of Medicine followed thirty-three overweight women through sixteen weeks of a structured cognitive-behavioral treatment program and then for one year after the program ended. The women lost an average of eighteen pounds during treatment, but more importantly, the group that reported relatively high activity levels after treatment fared far better than the least active group during the one-year follow-up. This more active one third of the participants, on average, achieved the goal of at least thirty minutes of activity per day at least five of seven days per week for 79 percent of the weeks during the follow-up year. This group continued losing weight during the follow-up period. This level of activity is close to the 12,000 steps per day goal. The least active third of the participants in the study achieved that goal during only 19 percent of the weeks in the follow-up period and on average they regained most of the weight that they had lost during treatment.
- **Simple:** Simple behavioral directives provide clear direction for actions, easily measured goals and readily available feedback about progress. Remember that wearing a pedometer provides great feedback, especially because feeling it on your hip or looking at the device over the course of the day helps remind you about your commitment. The direction for action and the goal are certainly clear and measurable: Walk enough to reach 12,000 steps on your pedometer every day.

- **Sustainable:** Walking is the preferred form of activity for most people. Young weight controllers in our Wellspring programs enjoy walking a lot more if their iPods or smart phones are attached to their ears. Walkers and runners actually move more and at higher intensities (faster) when listening to music. Many of our alumni families walk together, shop together and use this very natural form of movement to create a more active lifestyle.

SITTING VS. STANDING VS. MOVING

The following table also helps make the point about the critical role of steps. Look at the differences between "sitting or lying down" versus "standing quietly" versus "walking fast." Standing up expends 20 percent more energy than sitting down. Walking fast expends more than 300 percent more energy than sitting down.

Sitting vs. Standing vs. Moving—Calories Expended per Minute

Sitting or Lying Down	2.0 calories per minute
Standing quietly	2.4 calories per minute
Walking Fast (4 mph)	8.2 calories per minute
Running (9 min. mile)	17.6 calories per minute

Even shopping expends almost three times more energy as sitting, as long as you keep moving. (When you buy something, you still get the benefit of standing, a 20 percent boost in energy expenditure.)

Some adult weight controllers even purchase desks that allow them to stand up (e.g., drafting tables) just to get that extra 20 percent energy expenditure. It also helps to know how to equate activities and sports to steps. The next tables should be helpful:

Step Equivalents per Minute (Hierarchical)

Activity	Equivalent # of Steps Per Minute of Activity	Activity	Equivalent # of Steps Per Minute of Activity
Bowling	55	Shopping	60
Cycling (5 mph)	55	Walking (2 mph)	60
Dancing (slow)	55	Canoeing (2.5 mph)	70

Step 4—Use Movement to Level the Playing Field

Activity	Equivalent # of Steps Per Minute of Activity	Activity	Equivalent # of Steps Per Minute of Activity
Golfing (with cart)	70	Stair climbing	140
Volleyball (leisurely)	70	Aerobics step training (4" step)	145
Rowing (leisurely)	75	Badminton	150
Vacuuming	75	Roller skating (moderate)	150
Washing the car	75		
Window cleaning	75	Cross-country skiing (leisurely)	155
Painting	80	Gardening (heavy)	155
Walking (3 mph)	80	Hiking (no load)	155
Mopping	85	Stairmaster	160
Gardening (moderate)	90	Tennis (singles)	160
Housework	90	Water skiing	160
Table tennis	90	Ice skating (competitive)	170
Ice skating (leisurely)	95	Dancing (fast)	175
Dancing (non-contact)	100	Hiking (10 lb. load)	180
Golfing (no cart)	100	Rowing machine	180
Walking (4 mph)	100	Running (5 mph)	185
Waxing the car	100	Judo (competitive)	185
Tennis (doubles)	110	Aerobics (intense)	190
Aerobic dancing (low impact)	115	Scuba diving	190
Swimming (25 yards/min.)	120	Weight training (60 seconds b/w sets)	190
Volleyball game	120	Snow shoveling	195
Bicycling (10 mph)	125	Soccer (competitive)	195
Weight training (90 seconds b/w sets)	125	Cycling (12 mph)	200
		Elliptical machine (moderate)	200
Basketball (leisurely, non-game)	130	Racquetball	205
		Squash	205
Skiing (downhill)	130	Cross-country skiing (moderate)	220
Mowing lawn	135		
Scrubbing floor	140	Basketball (game)	220

Activity	Equivalent # of Steps Per Minute of Activity	Activity	Equivalent # of Steps Per Minute of Activity
Swimming (50 yards/min.)	225	Elliptical machine (fast)	270
Handball	230	Skipping rope	285
Jogging (6 mph)	230	Swimming (75 yards/min.)	290
Hiking (30 lb. load)	235	Running (8 mph)	305
Weight training (40 seconds b/w sets)	255	Cross-country skiing (fast)	330
		Running (10 mph)	350

STEP EQUIVALENTS PER MINUTE (ALPHABETICAL LISTING)

Activity	Equivalent # of Steps Per Minute of Activity	Activity	Equivalent # of Steps Per Minute of Activity
Aerobic dancing (low impact)	115	Cycling (12 mph)	200
		Cycling (5 mph)	55
Aerobics (intense)	190	Dancing (fast)	175
		Dancing (non-contact)	100
Aerobics step training (4" step)	145	Dancing (slow)	55
Badminton	150	Elliptical machine (fast)	270
Basketball (game)	220	Elliptical machine (moderate)	200
Basketball (leisurely, non-game)	130	Gardening (heavy)	155
Bicycling (10 mph)	125	Gardening (moderate)	90
Bowling	55	Golfing (no cart)	100
Canoeing (2.5 mph)	70	Golfing (with cart)	70
Cross-country skiing (fast)	330	Handball	230
Cross-country skiing (leisurely)	155	Hiking (10 lb. load)	180
Cross-country skiing (moderate)	220	Hiking (30 lb. load)	235

Step 4—Use Movement to Level the Playing Field

Activity	Equivalent # of Steps Per Minute of Activity	Activity	Equivalent # of Steps Per Minute of Activity
Hiking (no load)	155	Stair climbing	140
Housework	90	Stairmaster	160
Ice skating (competitive)	170	Swimming (25 yards/min.)	120
Ice skating (leisurely)	95	Swimming (50 yards/min.)	225
Jogging (6 mph)	230	Swimming (75 yards/min.)	290
Judo (competitive)	185	Table tennis	90
Mopping	85	Tennis (doubles)	110
Mowing lawn	135	Tennis (singles)	160
Painting	80	Vacuuming	75
Racquetball	205	Volleyball (leisurely)	70
Roller skating (moderate)	150	Volleyball game	120
Rowing (leisurely)	75	Walking (2 mph)	60
		Walking (3 mph)	80
Rowing machine	180	Walking (4 mph)	100
Running (10 mph)	350	Washing the car	75
		Water skiing	160
Running (5 mph)	185	Waxing the car	100
Running (8 mph)	305	Weight training (40 seconds b/w sets)	255
Scrubbing floor	140		
Scuba diving	190		
Shopping	60	Weight training (60 seconds b/w sets)	190
Skiing (downhill)	130		
Skipping rope	285	Weight training (90 seconds b/w sets)	125
Snow shoveling	195		
Soccer (competitive)	195		
		Window cleaning	75
Squash	205		

STRATEGIES FOR REACHING 12,000 STEPS

Get Up Early

Wellspring campers get their steps in a host of ways, but one key strategy involves getting up early. All campers are up at 7:00 a.m. so they can get in an hour of activity before breakfast. This may seem like something you'll want to skip at home. But think hard about this: early mornings are the only time of day we all can control.

Walk to Watch

One of the more noteworthy innovations at Wellspring's former boarding schools was the requirement that students had to be on a treadmill, elliptical or stationary bike in order to watch television programs. This will be too much for most families to enforce. However, I strongly recommend purchasing at least one piece of fitness equipment for the room where most television is watched. If you're buying one, consistent with our focus on walking, you'll do better with a treadmill—not an elliptical or a bike or some even fancier machine that claims it burns even more calories per minute of use. The key word in the last sentence is *use*: treadmills get used much more than other fitness equipment.

Putting a treadmill in front (hopefully directly in front) of the television is an important step for promoting activity. It helps to have many channels and the capability of watching movies in front of such machines.

GETTING STEPS IN MANY WAYS: DIMENSIONS OF MOVEMENT

Although getting 12,000 steps per day is the key to long-term weight control, it's also important to consider some other aspects of being active. At Wellspring, families ask some great questions about movement. Consider your answers to the following:

- Does it matter if my daughter does the same form of exercise every day?

- Isn't variety both the spice of life and the thing that helps kids stay motivated to stay active?
- Walking doesn't seem like real exercise to me. Don't you have to break a sweat to help you lose weight?
- I've heard many trainers talk about the value of taking a rest day at least once a week. How does that fit with the Wellspring Plan?

The American College of Sports Medicine (ACSM) has provided recommendations to answer these questions. ACSM consists of many of the world's leading experts on activity. ACSM's most recent set of recommendations has become accepted around the world as the basis for developing safe and effective activity patterns.

Let's review answers to commonly asked questions by considering five aspects of activity and the ACSM recommendations that pertain to each one. These aspects are:

- Frequency of activity
- Intensity of activity
- Duration of activity
- Variety of activity
- Strength training

Frequency of Activity

The Wellspring Plan goal is taking 12,000 steps every single day. Not every other day or even six days a week. Consistency can make a huge difference for weight controllers. You may recall that masters of weight control who participated in the National Weight Control Registry studies report about one hour's worth of brisk walking each day. These people know that activity every day helped them succeed.

In terms of biology, daily activity helps prevent the negative effects of what is sometimes called "the desert island effect" on metabolism. When weight controllers reduce food intake and lose weight, the body reacts by lowering the metabolic rate. The metabolic rate is the amount of energy our bodies expend to keep us alive at rest. This includes energy to keep the heart pumping and the liver working to break down the food we eat and transfer the energy from the food into our cells. Even active people expend more energy on these bodily functions operating twenty-four hours (86,400 seconds) per day than they expend for movement and exercise. So, metabolic rate matters a great deal. When the body detects a reduction in food intake, it "thinks" something like, *"Uh oh, I've got to conserve energy to keep this person alive."* Remember, humans survived as hunter-gatherers for tens of thousands of years, and evolution caused our bodies to adapt by lowering our metabolic rate when we had trouble finding enough food. This metabolic shift helped us survive much longer during famines. This is called the "desert island effect." If you found yourself abandoned on a desert island, this metabolic shift might save your life by allowing you to survive with relatively few calories.

Staying active every day allows weight controllers to reverse the desert island effect. The first study on this in 1984 showed that about thirty minutes of brisk walking can keep the metabolic rate in a normal range despite lowered caloric intake of food. This finding has been confirmed in many studies over the past thirty years. Our ability to reverse the desert island effect with activity only lasts about twenty-four hours. To keep the metabolic rate normal and make weight loss easier, weight controllers must stay active virtually every day, not just a few or even most days of the week.

Another important reason for the daily goal is that it is simpler, clearer, more difficult to rationalize non-compliance and much more effective. With a daily goal, it's hard to make excuses to avoid activity. This contrasts with a five-day-a-week goal, where most people will wind up saying to themselves: "Today is the day I won't exercise. I'll exercise tomorrow." This kind of thinking tends to result in skipping one day after another, and then abandonment.

Intensity of Activity

Intensity refers to how hard your body works over a period of time. More intensive activity means the body works harder for the fifteen or thirty or forty-five minutes when you're active. Intensity varies depending on one's level of conditioning or fitness. For example, world-class marathoners can run three eight-minute miles in a row without breaking a sweat. To the average person, this intensity would prove extremely challenging. The most important rule of thumb about intensity is: Keep the intensity low enough to allow yourself to be active comfortably for at least thirty minutes per session.

Duration of Activity

The ACSM endorses activity sessions lasting from 30 to 60 minutes. However, some overweight people have difficulty maintaining aerobic activity for 30 minutes or more. If this describes you, try starting with sessions that last 10 or 15 minutes. Two 15-minute sessions of exercise produce about the same benefits as one 30-minute session.

Some confusing notions exist about required duration of activity. One concerns "fat burning," suggesting you won't "burn fat" unless you're active for an extended period. This assertion is wrong. When you begin activity, you begin using calories immediately. Initially, the energy consumed by your body comes from glucose stored in the muscles. As you exercise for longer periods of time, your body begins dipping into its energy reserves (fat). However, your body must replenish the energy supply it uses. This means that when you consume energy in the form of stored glucose from the muscles, your body will use its stored energy supply to replenish the glucose taken from the muscles. It makes no difference whether you're active for short bursts of ten or fifteen minutes or for longer periods of thirty to sixty minutes per session. Both ways burn fat.

Duration can help you much more than intensity for weight control. Consider how to get the most steps. If you walk for an hour, you'll take between 6,000 and 8,000 steps. If you run as hard as you can for as long as you can for four minutes, you'll get about 1,000 steps. Keep this comparison in mind to remember that anything you do that involves movement of any kind works far better than doing very intense activities that can prove frustrating and exhausting.

Variety of Activity

Imagine what would happen if you fed your dog some brand new Super Chow. Assuming this dog chow tastes great—and because it's very low-fat, you can bet that it does—when you serve him the first bowl, he gobbles it down right away. Then he glances at you with those begging eyes hoping for another bowl. After a month or two, you notice that the Super Chow stays inside your dog's bowl for half the day, barely touched. He eats it eventually, but the gusto is gone. Then you switch him back to what he used to eat—Brand X. You're a bit surprised to see that your dog is chomping down on Brand X with the same gusto he used to have for Super Chow. After a month or so on Brand X, the dog's interest in this chow declines. The first day you re-introduce Super Chow, his gusto returns.

You've heard the expression "variety is the spice of life." So it is with your dog. And so it is with weight controllers, particularly novice weight controllers. In terms of getting 12,000 steps, variety adds excitement and increases the probability of achieving this important goal.

Strength Training (Weightlifting)

Beginning in 1990, ACSM recognized and emphasized the importance of resistance training more than in any of their previous recommendations. Strength training of moderate intensity (50 to 60 percent of your maximal lifting ability) provides important benefits. In particular, strength training can prevent injuries and reshape the body in favorable directions.

ACSM recommends selecting exercises that incorporate many different body parts and different kinds of movements. They suggest performing lifting exercises continuously, using smooth, slow and controlled motions. Maintaining a good posture while lifting also helps avoid injury. Only the body part being exercised while lifting the weight should be in motion during a lift. Other body parts should be at rest and stationary when weightlifting.

The following shows some frequently asked questions and answers about strength training.

Frequently Asked Questions about Strength Training

- *How many repetitions?* Eight to twelve repetitions improve both strength and endurance. Most exercise experts suggest that if you can lift the weight easily more than twelve times, it is time to add more weight. When you add more weight, go back to eight to twelve repetitions per exercise.
- *How many sets?* The ACSM recommends using eight to ten different kinds of weightlifting exercises per set. If you only make time to do one set, you will still strengthen your muscles 70 to 80 percent as much as you would by doing multiple sets. Two sets yields about 95 percent of the maximum benefit and three sets creates the full benefit or 100 percent. A full set of

eight or ten lifting exercises, including warm-up time, can take as little as fifteen minutes to do.

- *How many workouts?* The ideal strengthening program includes three workouts a week. Squeezing in more than three workouts per week might slow the growth of your muscles. Muscles may need some time off to recover from weight training. Interestingly, you can get about 75 percent of the maximum improvement available from weightlifting by working out only twice a week. If you don't have much time, even a single strengthening session per week helps far more than none at all. According to one study, a weekly workout can maintain current levels of strength for several months.
- *How much is enough?* To keep building strength, you must keep increasing the weights you lift. You can maintain a desired level of strength by simply maintaining twelve repetitions for a particular exercise. If you stop weightlifting, your strength will begin to fade within two weeks. After three to five months, you'll be back to where you started.
- *What's the procedure for weightlifting?* Several guidelines can help prevent injuries and maximize the benefits of weightlifting.
    1. It helps to warm up for a few minutes by walking briskly or jogging in place, and then doing stretching exercises. It helps to stretch your shoulders, lower back, calves and front and back of the thighs. Stretch slowly and steadily to the point of tension, not pain, and hold the position for three to thirty seconds.
    2. Breathe slowly and steadily during weightlifting. Holding your breath while tensing muscles can cause light-headedness and even fainting. Exhale as you either lift the weight or raise your body, and inhale as you return to the starting position.
    3. Perform the repetitions slowly. Each one should take about six seconds—two to lift and four to lower. Jerky movements can cause injury and soreness.
    4. Stop if your muscles hurt. The dictum "No pain, no gain" is both wrong and potentially dangerous. Your muscles should feel fatigued during the last repetitions, but you should

not feel sharp or piercing pains in your muscles. If you do feel pain, stop the exercise immediately.

5. Cool down after you exercise by doing a few minutes of walking or light jogging, followed by stretching again.

TAKING THE NEXT STEP: PLANNING

This plan was developed by one of my clients for a recent Thanksgiving break. Notice the level of detail and major facets of the plan, including a component focused on problem solving. The key is to focus on how to achieve 12,000+ steps—regardless of the time of year or obstacles in the way. Achieving this goal can take you a long way toward permanent success.

Goals and Plans for the Thanksgiving Break

1. STEPS PER DAY—GOALS:
    Minimum Level: 12,000
    Average: 15,000
   PLANS:
   - ✓ Morning mp3 player walk, 45 min.
   - ✓ Walk the dog in the evening—20 min.
   - ✓ Keep moving whenever possible.
   - ✓ No escalators or elevators when shopping.

2. WORKOUT ACTIVITIES—GOALS:
Bands every day; workouts two-four days
   PLANS:
   - ✓ YMCA with a friend at least once
   - ✓ YMCA total at least twice
   - ✓ Bands in the a.m. every day

3. MINIMIZING SEDENTARY BEHAVIORS—GOALS:
Three hours per day max on TV and computer

PLANS:
- ✓ I'll shop, bowl, whatever every day—be sure to hit my pedometer goals.

4. SOURCES OF ENCOURAGEMENT:
- ✓ I'll e-mail a friend at least once a day about how it's going.
- ✓ I'll bring the *Calorie King* book and read at least something in it every day.
- ✓ I'll talk a lot with my family about this.

5. METHODS OF PROBLEM SOLVING
- ✓ I'll self-monitor and journal every day.
- ✓ I'll be honest with myself if I get in trouble or really upset, then get consoled by a friend about it.

CHAPTER 9

Step 5—Develop an Athlete's Healthy Obsession

> **Persistence**
> Nothing in the world can take the place of persistence.
> Talent will not;
> nothing is more common than unsuccessful people with talent.
> Genius will not;
> unrewarded genius is almost a proverb.
> Education will not;
> the world is full of educated derelicts.
> Persistence and determination alone are omnipotent.
>
> — *Calvin Coolidge, 1932*

This perspective by President Coolidge hits upon a concept that rings true for every coach, every graduate admissions committee and most employers. These decision-makers all seek candidates who persist in the face of challenges. They aim to populate their teams, programs and companies with people who persist despite inevitable obstacles, almost regardless of innate talent.

Basketball great Ernie DiGregorio understood this when he was twelve years old: "Nobody gets up at six in the morning to play ball, but I did. At twelve years old, my mind was made up: I was going to play pro ball…I started practicing nine, ten hours a day by myself, with gloves, and I loved it. They could've cut my right hand off and I'd have played one-handed."

The "Great One," Wayne Gretzky, was renowned for his work ethic on and off the ice. Gretzky believed that, "The highest compliment that you can pay me is to say that I work hard every day, that I never dog it."

Most people know this innately: persistence wins in the end. But the question remains: How can I create this in myself or nurture it? This is exactly the purpose of the overarching mission in the Wellspring Plan, to develop a healthy obsession.

THE HEALTHY OBSESSION

Although the word obsession tends to have negative connotations in the outside world, in the Wellspring Plan I use the word "obsession" to refer to persistent thoughts that compel actions. If an obsession is healthy, it will help you achieve a positive way of living. For weight controllers, a healthy obsession is a very strong drive toward achieving the Wellspring Plan's three simple goals: eating very low-fat, getting 12,000 steps per day and self-monitoring 100 percent. A healthy obsession results in more daydreams, plans and routines that help maintain key behaviors. Remember, weight control is an athletic challenge—overcoming a biology that resists achievement of the goal. Also, our obesogenic culture makes it even harder to succeed. It's like trying to run a five-minute mile into a strong headwind. Our biology and the headwind never give us a break, nor do they give partial credit for moderate—albeit sincere—efforts.

It requires a great deal of persistence to become a successful weight controller. That's the healthy obsession—focusing the weight controller on consistency of eating, moving and self-monitoring—to overcome these barriers to success.

DEFINITION

A healthy obsession is a sustained preoccupation with the planning and execution of target behaviors to reach a healthy goal. Some other elements of the definition include aspects that are and are not defining characteristics of healthy obsessions.

A healthy obsession is:

- Knowing that your biology has turned against you and does not go on vacations or cut you slack because "you've had a rough day."
- Accepting the tough goal of eating as little fat as possible every day.

- Knowing that "the devil is in the details," so that writing down all food eaten is critical.
- Understanding that everything counts—everything.
- Being unwilling or very reluctant to accept permission, even from yourself, to overindulge.
- Making plans to help yourself stick with the Wellspring Plan at parties, restaurants and on trips.
- Analyzing lapses in order to prevent the same problem from happening tomorrow.
- Refusing to allow lapses to become relapses.
- Refusing to let a number on a scale prevent you from persisting.
- Feeling anxious if the three simple goals are not met.
- Accepting the idea that activity every day is the way, and doing it—even when you don't feel like it.
- Being an active problem solver, oriented to take action, not just to analyze.

A healthy obsession is NOT:

- Seeking moderation in all things.
- Giving yourself permission to deviate from the program because of moods, stress, holidays or vacations.
- Waltzing into a high-risk situation (like a party or a cafeteria) without a plan.
- Making lame excuses for major lapses.
- Allowing lapses to turn into relapses.
- Feeling just fine when goals are sometimes not met.
- Getting thrown into a major tailspin because a number on a scale is too high.
- Wallowing in self-pity.
- Getting discouraged and overwhelmed.

A HEALTHY OBSESSION STARTS WITH SELF-MONITORING

Every diet requires some change in eating patterns and a reduction in calories consumed. But diets also give weight controllers hope and—even more important—increase awareness. The most helpful aspects of any diet lie in these factors, not in the magic of grapefruit or the latest ideas in combining foods. Self-monitoring can create that awareness better than any other behavioral strategy.

> **The key behavioral component for successful long-term weight control is self-monitoring, the systematic observation of key behaviors (eating and moving) and the recording of those observations.**

A person who wishes to change himself should demand an account of himself with regard to the particular point which he has resolved to watch in order to correct himself and improve. Let him go over the single hours or periods from the time he arose to the hour and moment of the present examination and make a mark for each time he has fallen into the particular sin or defect. The second day should be compared with the first, that is, the two examinations of the present day with the two of the preceding day. Let him observe if there is an improvement from one day to another. Let him compare one week with another and observe whether he has improved during the present week as compared to the preceding.

— St. Ignatius Loyola, 1500

St. Ignatius Loyola's thoughts on behavioral change date from the middle ages but are very accurate, based on current scientific knowledge. Researchers have demonstrated the importance of self-monitoring to improve performance across a wide range of disciplines. Self-monitoring is used extensively in sports. Professional football players want to know how fast they run the forty-yard dash. Pitchers want to know how fast and how accurately they are pitching. Feedback is the key ingredient for improved performance. In one famous study, Olympic-level figure skaters were left to train on their own. They attempted sixty elements (jumps, spins) in an hour of training. Then, a whiteboard was brought out onto the ice so their coach could tally the number of jumps and spins in real time. The result: the number of elements attempted rose from sixty to one hundred. Then the whiteboard was removed, and the number declined to sixty. Then the coach brought the whiteboard out again. The result: suddenly the figure skaters were attempting one hundred elements again.

Many scientific studies have demonstrated the importance of self-monitoring for successful long-term weight control. Simply put, weight controllers who self-monitor consistently lose much more weight and keep if off much better than those who don't self-monitor consistently. Leading obesity researcher Tom Wadden of the University of Pennsylvania described self-monitoring as the "cornerstone" of behavioral treatment for weight problems.

What is Self-Monitoring? For the past ten years, participants in Wellspring's programs used small booklets as their self-monitoring journals or SMJs:

Here's how participants in Wellspring use their SMJs: At the beginning of each day, they circle the day of the week and write down the date. Then, at breakfast, they write down everything they eat. This includes:

- What you're eating
- Portion size (# of ounces or cups)
- Calories
- Fat grams

They repeat the process for lunch, dinner and snacks. They're advised to write down something—anything—that occurs to them in the "Think and Ink" section. This section comprises a journaling technique. Journaling, just writing down thoughts and feelings without focusing on the quality of the writing, can improve focusing, manage moods and promote success in various tasks. The "Link" section allows the weight controller to extract key thoughts or ideas about the day.

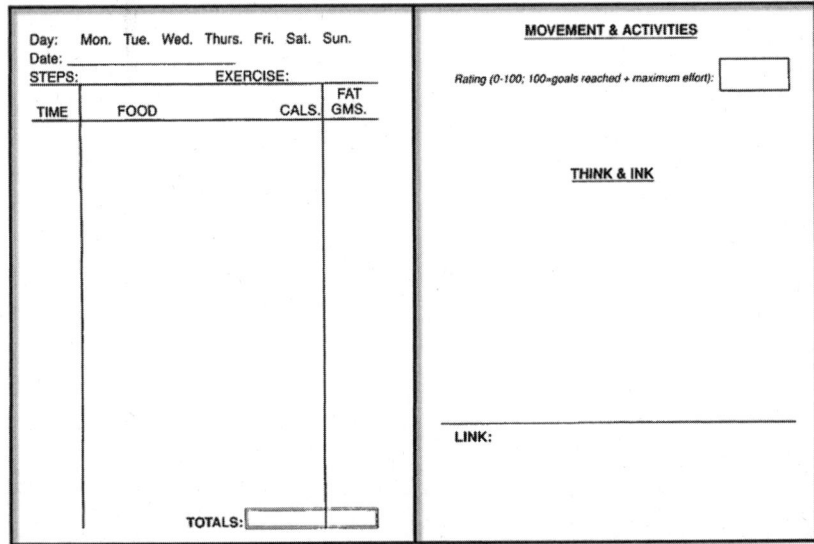

At the end of the day, participants in these programs:
- Recorded steps where it says STEPS (top left).
- Totaled their calories and fat grams for the day.
- Reviewed how active they were—on a scale of 1 to 100 with 100 being as active as you possibly could be, was today a 20 or an 80 (top right of the second page)?

You may be wondering: how will I know how many calories or fat grams are in a particular food? Wellspring participants use a wonderful pocket-sized book mentioned in the food chapter called *The CalorieKing Calorie, Fat and Carbohydrate Counter* (written by dietitian Allan Borushek and updated annually). This book is also available online and as an app for smart phones, as are other calorie and fat counters.

Why is Self-Monitoring So Important?

Wellspring campers have had a lot to say about self-monitoring's value. Here are some of their comments:
- "Self-monitoring keeps me from lying to myself."
- "Self-monitoring helps me stay mindful of what I'm eating."
- "Self-monitoring makes me knowledgeable about what I'm doing and keeps me connected to my goal of weight control."
- "Self-monitoring helps me solve problems and make adjustments in order to stay successful."
- "Self-monitoring keeps me from feeling ashamed about what I eat. This helps keep some of the emotion out of eating and helps me stay more objective and focused on problem-solving in order to succeed."
- "Self-monitoring helps me cope and helps me feel in control."
- "Self-monitoring helps me appreciate challenges like new restaurants. It is also the key to weight loss: being self-aware."
- "Keeping track in my head doesn't work nearly as well as self-monitoring on paper."

These great observations identified most of the mechanisms which make self-monitoring the key to long-term weight control. It helps people maximize their commitment to their goals, stay committed to them, feel in control, understand their patterns of eating and moving, focus on the details and even keep their moods more positive. The next summary provides a quick review of these points.

Why Self-Monitoring Helps

Consistent self-monitoring improves weight control by:

- Increasing ability to use GOALS
- Strengthening COMMITMENT to change
- Increasing coping and feelings of CONTROL
- Improving understanding of EATING/EXERCISE PATTERNS
- Promoting more POSITIVE MOODS
- Improving information about, and focusing on, the DETAILS

The experiences of participants in these programs strongly suggest the power of self-monitoring. Decades of scientific research confirm its importance.

Science Supports the Value of Self-monitoring. No researcher or healthcare professional familiar with the scientific literature on weight control would disagree with the value of self-monitoring. Table 9-1 shows some of the findings from studies on this very point. The results demonstrate that when people write down at least 75 percent of their eating and exercising behaviors, they are much more likely to be successful in losing weight and maintaining weight loss. Failing to write down these critical aspects of weight control tends to result in minimal or temporary success.

Table 9-1
Research on the Benefits of Consistent Self-Monitoring

- At our Wellspring Camps, we found that campers who self-monitored most consistently during camp were more than twice as likely as those who monitored less consistently to lose clinically significant amounts of weight during a six to nine-month follow-up period. The next figure illustrates this finding.
- Among weight controllers in a twelve-week program, those who self-monitored consistently lost 64 percent more weight than the inconsistent self-monitors. Consistent self-monitors also maintained this superior weight loss three months later.
- Weight controllers who discontinued self-monitoring during the holiday season (Thanksgiving to New Year's Day) gained

fifty-seven times more weight than their counterparts who continued to self-monitor consistently.
- Two studies showed that even weight controllers who self-monitor very consistently often discontinue monitoring for a day or more. During the weeks when they took a day or more "off," they lost much less weight than usual. Specifically, when these consistent self-monitors kept track of virtually everything they ate and all of their activity, they lost between one and two pounds per week. In contrast, during their least consistent weeks, they lost only half as much weight.
- Weight controllers who were generally inconsistent self-monitors gained an average of one pound per week during their least consistent self-monitoring weeks. They fared much better—in fact they maintained their weight—during weeks in which they self-monitored almost every day.
- In two different studies, only highly consistent self-monitors lost weight during the holiday season (Thanksgiving to New Year's).
- Weight controllers who self-monitored very consistently in the first few weeks of several outpatient professional treatment programs maintained much greater weight losses, compared to inconsistent self-monitors, when evaluated one to two years after treatment began.
- In two follow-up studies conducted one to one-and-a-half years after participants completed their stays in one of our Wellspring Camps, we found that highly successful campers used self-monitoring far more often than unsuccessful campers.

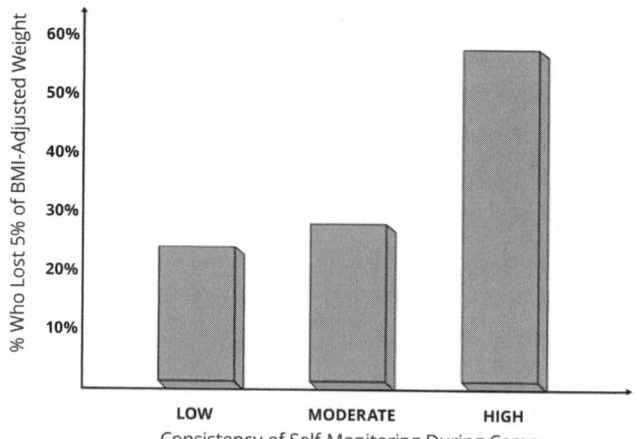

Does it Matter How You Monitor?

Probably not. Many weight controllers use online programs or phone apps and the research indicates that consistency matters a lot, but not the format of self-monitoring. So, this very simple saying can help you review the kind of focus that self-monitoring helps generate:

Everything Counts!

Weight control does not begin on a Monday or on the first day of a new month or on the first day of a new year. It begins as soon as weight controllers make a sincere effort to control eating and moving. By making everything count, self-monitoring helps create the foundation for the broader concept, the key attitude and approach, defined by the term "healthy obsession."

THE SCIENCE OF THE HEALTHY OBSESSION

Decades of research strongly suggest the benefits of a healthy obsession for successful long-term weight control. The following points summarize some of the more compelling findings:

- Perhaps the most consistent finding over the past thirty years in weight-loss literature is that when weight controllers regularly attend professionally conducted weight loss therapy, they usually persist and succeed at losing weight almost every week. Two studies randomly assigned people to groups in which they received either long-term or short-term professional behavioral weight-loss therapy. In both studies, the groups that received a longer course of treatment lost far more weight. Attending weekly sessions helps people focus on the details of their eating, greatly increases their consistency of self-monitoring and promotes the development of a healthy obsession (e.g., more planning and problem solving).
- In a series of studies, psychologist Michael Perri and his colleagues from the University of Florida found that almost any effort that consistently focused the attention of their clients on the process of losing weight improved maintenance of weight loss. Comparing different types of booster sessions held weekly over six months, the researchers found that sessions

focused on relapse prevention or problem solving did not help maintain weight losses any better than those focused on very general discussions of recipes and other weight-loss issues. The conclusion: Any kind of contact—even sending postcards or making brief phone calls, regardless of the content—improved the ability of weight controllers to maintain weight loss as compared to people who did not receive such attention. Attention from concerned others leads to more intensive focus on goals, plans and commitments (i.e., healthy obsessions).

- The National Weight Control Registry includes responses to surveys by more than two thousand people who have lost, on average, fifty pounds and kept it off for six years. On average, these master long-term weight controllers (LTWCs) lost and regained 270 pounds before they were finally successful. Another survey of two hundred LTWCs found that final success came only after an average of five previous temporarily successful weight losses. The reason they finally succeeded? A much more intensive approach. In fact, the majority of LTWCs in the National Weight Control Registry used a much stricter dietary regimen (very low-fat) and more than 80 percent reported they exercised far more than in previous attempts. They also reported paying much more careful attention to their weight, their eating and activity.

- Another study by Michael Perri and his colleagues focused on 379 sedentary adults who wanted to become more active and fit. Half of the participants were asked to walk for thirty minutes three to four days per week (moderate approach) while the other half was asked to walk for the same duration five to seven days per week (intensive approach). The researchers expected the moderate approach to result in more walking than the intensive approach over time. The healthy obsession concept would argue that daily activity improves focus and leads to more consistent activity over the long haul. In fact, over a six-month period, the more intensive approach led to 53 percent more walking than the moderate approach.

- A study by psychologist Eric Stice of Stanford University makes a related point about dieting. Dr. Stice followed a large sample of teens ages sixteen to nineteen over nine months. Dr. Stice found that many were dieting to some extent. The most important finding from this study is that moderate levels of dieting were associated with weight *gain* while more intensive forms were associated with weight *loss*. Dr. Stice's intensive dieters, for example, regularly used eighteen out of nineteen possible dietary behaviors in order to try to lose weight. Moderate dieters reported using only half of these dietary behaviors.

- Wellspring researchers conducted two studies involving intensive interviews with either very successful or unsuccessful campers more than a year post-camp. These studies involved asking a series of probing questions about healthy obsessions using the "Wellspring Transformative Change Interview." In one of those recent studies, Kristen Gierut and I found both numerical (quantitative) and qualitative differences between the successful weight controllers (named "Losers" in this study) and unsuccessful weight controllers ("Gainers"). Here's how we summarized those differences:

Quantitative Differentiators

You're on vacation with your family for ten days. On how many of those days would you eat twenty grams of fat or less? Losers reported they would eat less than 20g of fat per day on almost twice as many days on that vacation than Gainers (M = 6.38 vs. 3.44 days).

You have three major exams coming up at school this week. You have to meet with groups, cram/study very hard and you feel very stressed about getting everything done and doing well. Of the seven days leading up to the exam, how many days would you monitor food? How many days would you get 10,000 steps? How many days would you eat 20g of fat or less? Losers reported they would continue to self-monitor an average of 5.25 days leading up to the exam vs. 3.94 days by Gainers. Losers indicated they would exercise on average 4.94 days leading up to the exam compared to 3.38 days by the Gainers. Losers also reported they would eat less than 20g of fat per day on an average of 5.88 days leading up to the exam vs. 4.69 days by Gainers.

You get into a fight with your best friend (boyfriend/girlfriend), and he/she does not speak to you for the rest of the day. Will you still eat less than 20 g of fat on this day? All Losers (8/8) reported they would still eat less than 20g of fat on this day whereas only half of the Gainers (4/8) reported they would still eat less than 20g of fat on this day.

You are heading to your friend's house for a party. You know that the food there will primarily consist of high-fat pizza and chips. Will you still reach your 10,000 step goal today? Will you still eat less than 20 g of fat this day? All Losers (8/8) indicated they would still reach their step goal vs. 5/8 of the Gainers (5/8). Similarly, all Losers (8/8) reported they would still eat less than 20g of fat on this day whereas only 5/8 of the Gainers reported they would eat within that key guideline of the Wellspring Plan.

Qualitative Differentiators

Let's imagine that you normally get in 10,000 steps every day by walking, but today your ankle really hurts; you injured it playing soccer yesterday, and it is uncomfortable to walk. Will this impact the food you eat this day? Only Losers demonstrated attitudes consistent with a healthy obsession by noting that they would decrease their eating because they expected the injury to prevent them from reaching their activity goals. In sharp contrast, two of the Gainers noted that they expected to overeat in response to the injury, not decrease their eating.

One Loser stated, "Yes, it would [impact the food I eat]. You have to change your diet since you'll do less exercise. You still need to lose weight that day." Another Loser mentioned, "I would make sure I'm being very careful of what I'm eating because I cannot meet my step goal." In contrast, a Gainer stated, "Probably [it would impact the food I eat] more in a negative way. I would probably feel sorry for myself. I would be less likely to get up and cook things because my ankle would hurt and to go out and get healthy things is unlikely if I'm injured." Another Gainer stated, "Um, I do find myself getting bored in situations like this and then I'd just eat more."

You get into a fight with your best friend (boyfriend/girlfriend), and he/she does not speak to you for the rest of the day. How does this impact your activity for the day? Losers again demonstrated more substantial healthy obsessions than Gainers. Losers reported that the fight with their friend would not impact their weight control programs whereas Gainers expected negative outcomes. One Loser stated, "I'll suck it up and do what I need to do. It wouldn't affect me." Similarly, another Loser reported, "It [the fight with a friend] doesn't impact my activity; well, to me that's a non-related event. You must exercise and you cannot let things hinder you." In contrast a Gainer stated, "Um, I'd sit there eating frozen yogurt and watch TV and cry. It affects me very much when I get into an argument." Another Gainer mentioned, "lower it [my activity] dramatically."

You are heading to your friend's house for a party. You know that the food there will primarily consist of high-fat pizza and chips. Do you have a plan for eating at the party? Losers used more definitive language about their plans, whereas Gainers used language such as "probably" and "I guess," illustrating less confidence in their responses. For example, one Loser stated, "Yes [I have a plan]. I'll bring a [fat-free snack]. I don't care what people say."

Another Loser stated, "Yes, I would eat before. It's a little trick that I do, because if you are already full you are not going to eat anything else. And just be like 'oh, no I am not hungry, thank you.' I would definitely eat before and make sure that it was fulfilling food so that I am satisfied." In contrast, a Gainer predicted, "Probably eat one plate and a few chips and go hang out."

Many other studies in peer-reviewed journals support the healthy obsession concept. We know, for example, that weight controllers who have greater stability in their lives because of their jobs, financial situations and mental health succeed more often than those with unstable personal and work situations. Some studies even find that older adults—those over sixty—tend to succeed more in professional weight loss programs than younger adults. One strong hypothesis is that greater stability in life allows weight controllers to focus more clearly on developing consistent patterns, a key element in healthy obsessions.

NURTURING A HEALTHY OBSESSION

Self-monitoring very consistently provides the most direct route to developing a healthy obsession. This chapter documented how powerfully both self-monitoring and healthy obsessions can impact success. Keeping the three primary behavioral goals in mind from the Wellspring Plan also reinforces the value of this approach (0 fat g; 12,000 steps; 100 percent self-monitoring). The image that follows illustrates the key point about healthy obsessions: It's fundamentally a choice in life. You either go down the road toward this challenging but rewarding way of living or you go on the other side (and therefore fail to achieve your weight loss goals). Just as serious athletes must make substantial commitments to their sports every day, so do weight controllers.

Another direction for nurturing your own healthy obsession comes from those around you and the environments in which you live and work every day. Very few athletes excel on their own, without encouragement and support from coaches, team mates and others. The next chapter focuses on how to build that winning team for your weight-controlling efforts.

Make Your Choice - Don't Look Back

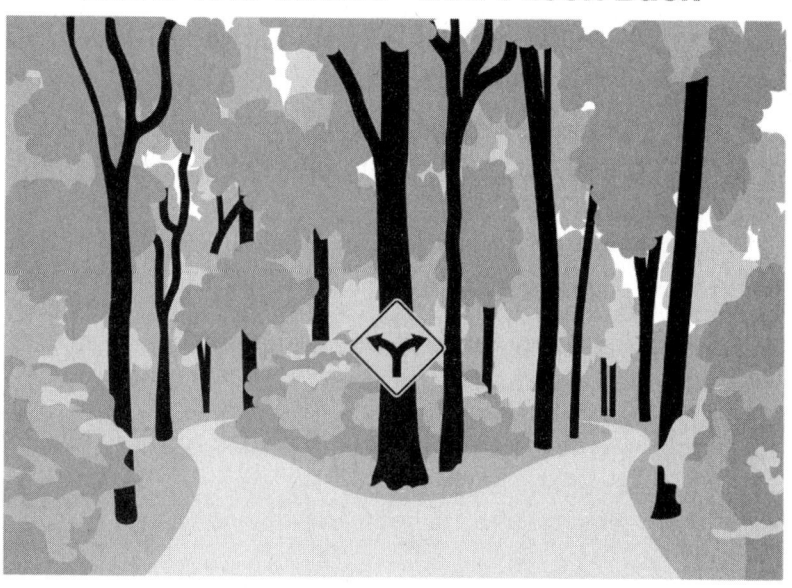

CHAPTER 10

Step 6—Build a Winning Team Around You

People with strong relationships suffer fewer medical and emotional problems than those who are more isolated. A study of seven thousand adults in California showed that people who lacked strong relationships with others died at a younger age than those who had strong relationships (i.e., married, made frequent contacts with friends and neighbors or belonged to social clubs or religious groups).

Many other studies demonstrate that support from others can reduce the effects of stressors:

- Women who have a companion with them during labor and childbirth experience fewer complications than women who give birth alone. Women in the supported group give birth sooner, are awake more after delivery and play more with their babies.
- Social support helps men who lose their jobs. Men with good support report fewer illnesses and less depression than men who do not have adequate support.
- Recovery from heart attacks is improved with the support of spouses, friends and relatives.
- Parents who receive training on parenting techniques and problem solving help their children lose more weight than those who do not.

We do better at almost anything when we're surrounded by people who actively show they care about us.

Most athletes certainly know this. Elite athletes build their own teams—even in individual pursuits—including personal coaches, trainers, sports psychologists and managers. Let's consider the types of support available to you, the types of coaches athletes seek and what you can do to create your best winning team.

TYPES OF SUPPORT

You can benefit from three types of support: emotional, informational and material.

Emotional Support

Others provide emotional support to you when they:

- Listen and talk things over with you, showing you understanding or empathy
- Show confidence in you and provide encouragement

Informational Support

People provide you with informational support when they:

- Give you worthwhile advice
- Provide you with resources that prove useful
- Suggest various solutions to problems from which you can choose courses of action

Material Support

You may receive material support from others sometimes in the form of:

- Food
- Money
- Shelter
- Clothing
- Education

Because the support of friends and family can play such an important role in managing the challenges of life, one great stress management

Exercise 10-1
Sources of Support in My Life

Instructions: *Fill in the blanks and see who emerges as your supportive friends, colleagues and family members.*

People who...	At Home	At Work	At Play
Calm me			
Bring me joy			
Make me laugh			
Listen to me			
Really care about me			
Provide me with material support when requested			
Challenge me, but in a good way			
Help me think through possible solutions to problems			
Energize me			
Seem to know amazing amounts of information			

skill is knowing when and whom to ask for help. Complete Exercise 10-1 to focus on those whom you can rely on to help you manage the challenges you face in your life.

Some of these supportive people in your life might want advice about how to support you most effectively. You can show them the suggestions in Table 10-1 to guide them.

Table 10-1
How to Support A Weight Controller's Efforts

Losing weight and keeping it off is a very difficult process. You can make it easier for your spouse, friend or partner. Here are several suggestions that will help you support and encourage the weight controllers in your life.

General Attitude

- *Be positive.* Convey to the weight controller that even though it is very difficult to control weight, you believe he or she can do it. This attitude will boost the person's self-confidence while acknowledging the difficulties. Avoid negative comments, criticism and coercion. These are unhelpful and demoralizing, and will create negative feelings between you and the weight controller. This, in turn, could cause him or her to eat more—not less—and thwart the likelihood of success in the long run.
- *Be reinforcing.* Acknowledge the weight controller's accomplishments. Compliments, attention, encouragement and tangible reinforcement (like little gifts) can help him or her stay motivated and adhere to the plan. Remember, be sincere; superficiality will be interpreted as condescending and aversive.
- *Be realistic.* Weight control requires tremendous effort and skill to overcome strong biological forces. People who are trying to lose weight must adopt eating and exercise patterns that are much more stringent than normal. Don't expect the weight controller to be perfect, or even close to perfect. Occasional slips of overeating, inactivity, weight gain and failure to adhere to plans will occur. Help the weight controller learn from these experiences rather than dwell on them as "failures."
- *Communicate.* Inquire occasionally about the weight controller's progress. Ask him or her how you can help, thereby complimenting the weight controller's individual efforts. Be open to discussing the challenges of weight control and to assisting in problem solving.

Managing Food

- Increase the amount of nutritious, low-fat foods available to the weight controller.
- Do NOT encourage the weight controller to eat foods that he or she is trying to avoid (for example, refrain from saying, "Let's go out for ice cream," or "Oh, come on, a little bit isn't going to hurt you.").

- Help the weight controller prepare foods and recipes in a low-fat way. Encourage experimentation and adventure.
- Adopt appropriate eating habits, for example: not eating when full, eating appropriate portions, eating in a slow, deliberate fashion, eating regularly or on a schedule, limiting snacking and limiting the number of eating situations. You may not have a weight problem, but better eating habits may improve your health and will support the weight controller's efforts.
- Plan activities with the weight controller that do not revolve around food (for example, sporting events, concerts, games).
- When you go to a restaurant with the weight controller, select places that make low-fat/low-sugar eating as pleasant as possible.

Promoting Exercise

- Plan activities with the weight controller that involve exercise (for example, walking, hiking, sports).
- Become an exercise partner. You will reap the same physical benefits as your partner.
- Support and encourage the weight controller's individual efforts to exercise.

TYPES OF COACHES: LESSONS LEARNED BY ATHLETES

Legendary UCLA basketball coach John Wooden, the "Wizard of Westwood," won an unprecedented ten NCAA basketball championships in twelve years. He emphasized effort more than winning and support/encouragement more than control:

"You cannot find a player who ever played for me who can tell you that he ever heard me mention winning a basketball game...The last thing that I told my players, just prior to tipoff, [was] 'When the game is over, I want your head up—and I know of only one way for your head to be up—and that's for you to know that you did your best...this means to do the best YOU can do. That's the best; no one can do more...you made that effort."

Very few coaches produce the kind of loyalty and intense admiration that virtually all of his players had for John Wooden. Very few athletes have a chance to play with such a legendary coach. But athletes often have choices about their coaches. What do they look for in a coach? How do the best coaches help their athletes? Research on coaching styles, athlete preferences and effective coaching techniques provide answers to these important questions.

COACHING STYLES

Research has identified three types of coaching styles. As you review them, consider which one you might prefer in someone who could help you as a trainer or weight control counselor.

Task-oriented vs. Relationship-oriented

Task-oriented coaches work together with athletes to get the job done. They focus on training and instruction. They attempt to improve the performances of their athletes by providing good technical instruction on skills, techniques and strategies. They emphasize and facilitate rigorous training. When players make errors, they focus on corrective, technical advice.

Relationship-oriented coaches focus more on developing interpersonal relationships between themselves and their athletes and within teams. They keep lines of communication open and maintain positivity in their connections to their athletes. They focus on how athletes feel, concentrating more on feelings and team spirit than on technical aspects of their sports.

Democratic vs. Autocratic

A democratic decision-making style allows athletes to participate in decisions. These types of coaches sometimes have athletes help decide about the team's goals, practice techniques and schedules and game plans—to varying extents. In contrast, the autocratically oriented coach remains aloof from athletes. These coaches stress their authority in making the team work and tend to seem powerful and intimidating.

Supportive vs. Punitive

Coaches who focus on support show concern for the welfare of each of their athletes. They attempt to establish warm, personal relationships with fewer boundaries off the playing field than most other types of coaches. They also emphasize the good in their athletes via positive reinforcement whenever possible. In contrast, some coaches use a punitive style which involves more critical comments and harshness toward the players. These coaches maintain rigid boundaries off the field. Perhaps the idea behind this emphasis is "spare the rod and spoil the child."

Most athletes prefer more supportive and democratic coaching styles. However, circumstances can significantly affect these preferences. For instance, as athletes get older and develop higher levels of skill, they tend to prefer more task-oriented and autocratic coaching styles. Also, athletes who themselves are more social and relationship oriented tend to perform better with coaches who emphasize such things. Another very logical differentiator pertains to the nature of the sport. Athletes who play large-scale, complex team sports like football and volleyball tend to prefer more autocratic styles than athletes who play individual sports like golf or bowling or tennis. This makes sense. More autocratic styles create more efficient and focused leadership. A democratic style in a highly complex team sport can cause confusion.

Lessons Learned

In addition to the pattern of preferences for coaches of different styles, athletes look for effectiveness of the coach. They want coaches who win. Winning coaches succeed because of skills in recruitment, reputation and knowledge of the sport and how best to teach and execute.

For weight controllers, some parallels in understanding could help you achieve your goals. For example, you can rely on measures of effectiveness just as athletes do. In your case, you'd want to get involved with programs and people who have demonstrated their effectiveness. Those demonstrations appear in scientific journals and reputations among respected professional referral sources. When you decide to attend programs or seek professional help, the following section will provide some useful guidance. You would also want to select leaders of the programs or consultation to match your knowledge and skill level as a weight controller. For example, if you've tried Weight Watchers several times before, you're not likely to find that useful at this stage in your program. More individualized consultation from higher-level experts or programs would suit you better, just as more experienced athletes prefer different coaching styles from their inexperienced peers.

CREATING YOUR TEAM: STRUCTURE WORKS

Athletes frequently develop structure around them, essentially their own teams. Team members include coaches, training buddies, personal trainers (strength, conditioning, sport-specific) and sometimes sport psychologists. They rely on these teams to keep them focused, exactly what weight controllers struggle to maintain quite often. Studies of sports psychology and weight management show that tremendous benefits accrue by adding effective, supportive teams around both athletes and weight controllers. Adding structure can range from simple changes to substantial and potentially more powerful interventions. Let's consider the major options in choosing your team for weight control.

Get a Little Help from Your Friends

Supportive friends can help you by working out with you, staying on the Wellspring Plan themselves, supporting you when you eat on plan, helping you problem solve if you hit a rough patch and in many other ways. These friends also stand to benefit by helping you. Many people want to increase their thinness and fitness. You can show them how to reach those goals as they help you reach yours.

Other Structured Assists

Personal trainers can help you stay focused and motivated. Most health clubs will only hire people with certifications from various recognized organizations, like the American Council of Sports Medicine (ASCM) and the American Council on Exercise (ACE). It's important to discuss your approach to eating with trainers. Many will have ideas other than those presented in this book. If your potential trainer objects to a very low-fat diet, for example, you can find another trainer.

Many other activities provide useful structure, too. For example, getting involved in community theater does not, at first blush, sound very active. Yet, that involvement can get you out of the house and moving. More directly active recreational sports, like city league volleyball or softball works great, as does joining a bowling league.

Join a Self-Help Group

This is an excellent way to add structure and remain focused on your goals. There are two well-known and widely available self-help groups in the US and Canada, with a worldwide presence for Weight Watchers as well as online assistance:

Take Off Pounds Sensibly (TOPS)

Founded in 1948, TOPS has two hundred thousand members and ten thousand chapters operating in the US, Canada and several other countries. To find the group meeting nearest you, go to **www.tops.org**, click on "Find a Meeting" and enter your zip code. I did this and found several chapters within ten miles of my home. Each chapter lists its meeting address and time, as well as the names of chapter leaders with phone numbers. Many chapters welcome teenagers and many Wellspring alumni have benefited from attending TOPS meetings to stay on program.

TOPS focuses on self-monitoring, healthful eating and staying active in a fashion consistent with the principles of Wellspring. While TOPS doesn't advocate a very low-fat approach or the use of pedometers and the 10,000-step goal, it can still be very useful to keep your weight controller focused and motivated. The cost is also low. You will have to become a member and pay nominal chapter fees (each chapter sets its own fees to cover operating expenses).

Weight Watchers

The only other non-professional approach that follows enough of the science of weight loss to warrant recommendation is Weight Watchers. Weight Watchers also encourages healthful eating and self-monitoring. There are over twenty thousand Weight Watchers groups around the country. To find a meeting, go to **www.weightwatchers.com** and click on "Find a Meeting." Weight Watchers also provides an extensive and somewhat interactive online program, advertised very heavily. However, research shows that actually attending group meetings produces much better results than the online program. Online programs simply do not engage participants very effectively; at least that's the result for the vast majority of people.

Although Weight Watchers is famous for its "Points" program, Weight Watchers also offers a "Core Program" that doesn't use points, but rather focuses on self-monitoring, education and support. I suggest you use the weekly meetings as an opportunity to improve your focus and commitment.

Other Self-help Approaches

Some other non-professional approaches, I believe, have numerous flaws from a scientific perspective. I don't recommend any other non-professional approach aside from TOPS and Weight Watchers for this reason.

Get Help from a Professional

Many hospitals and medical centers offer professional weight management programs that can help some people achieve greater success than non-professional self-help programs. Look for programs directed by psychologists or other mental health professionals with expertise in cognitive-behavioral therapy, the approach that has the best track record by far and forms the basis of much of the Wellspring Plan. The better weight management programs are open-ended, providing help for unlimited periods of time and definitely no less than one year. Longer term programs tend to produce better outcomes.

These three organizations also have listings of mental health professionals in virtually every area of the United States:

1) **Association for Advancement of Behavioral and Cognitive Therapies**
    Go to **www.abct.org** and click on "Find a therapist."
2) **American Psychological Association**
    Go to **www.apa.org** and click on "Find a psychologist."
3) **National Association of Social Workers**
    Go to **www.helpstartshere.org** and click on "Find a social worker."

Calls to local hospitals and to the psychology departments of local colleges and universities may prove helpful, too.

Immersion Programs

Programs like Wellspring Camps immerse weight controllers in a structured world of healthy living and provide them with education, encouragement and cognitive-behavioral therapy to help them change. Wellspring provides immersion for adults as well as teenagers. This intensive experience typically results in rapid weight loss and builds tremendous momentum to develop a healthy obsession.

Participating in immersion programs can help you experience genuine success, and success really can promote more of the same. It's unfortunate that it is so challenging to compete with the biological and environmental challenges that resist weight loss. So it's certainly possible that you may not be able to overcome these barriers even with help from professionals dedicated to the same scientific principles as those described in this book. If this is the case, a scientifically based immersion program can make a huge difference. Immersion can also solidify and strengthen commitment.

CHAPTER 11

Step 7—Become Undisturbable

Consider these two athletic situations then compare them to weight control. Try to find commonalities between the athletic and weight control situations.

ATHLETIC SITUATION 1: PRESSURE ON THE PITCHER

JJ, a pitcher, has thrown the ball very well deep into the game. It's a very hot day in Atlanta, steamy and in the high nineties. JJ feels weak going into the eighth inning, with the score tied 2-2. He is still throwing well, but his teammates have just made two fielding errors, putting men at first and second. Then JJ throws an inside fastball and barely nicks the arm of the batter. It looked like the batter leaned in to get hit. An argument ensues. Now, JJ is feeling really hot and tired and the bases are full. Where does he get the strength to stay focused and go after that last batter for the inning?

ATHLETIC SITUATION 2: DISTRACTED HIGH SCHOOL SWIMMER

Competing in the individual medley for her high school's swim team has been Kristen's dream since she started swimming as a preschooler. Her mother and older sister swam for the same high school and Kristen was eager to keep that family tradition very much alive. The practice schedule demanded a great deal from the swimmers: practicing in the pool for one-and-a-half hours before school and another hour plus after school every weekday, plus competitions on Saturdays. Kristen started struggling with her academic studies in school, which bothered her a lot, and then her boyfriend of two years broke up with her. Kristen became so distracted that she didn't go to practice for two days. Her coach threatened to bench her for a month. How does Kristen get the strength to focus on her swimming again?

WEIGHT CONTROLLER ON A SINKING SHIP

Mike had thoroughly bought into the Wellspring Plan. His wife and two teenage children embraced the approach as well. He managed to self-monitor consistently, eat very little fat and average 14,000 steps per day. He lost twenty-five of the sixty pounds he wanted to lose in three months. In addition to working hard at his full-time job, Mike paid close attention to his aging mother, who was barely hanging on to her independence in a retirement community about thirty minutes from Mike's house. Then in the course of two weeks, Mike lost his job and his mother became seriously ill. Mike began missing some days of self-monitoring and failing to get his steps beyond about 6,000. Where does Mike get the strength to right the sinking weight control ship?

Each scenario ended by asking a question about strength. Demands from within the athletic arena affected JJ, the baseball player; challenges from school and a break-up distracted Kristen, the swimmer; and Mike, the weight controller, experienced major changes in his mother's health and his employment.

Respected psychologists Roy Baumeister and Todd Heatherton define these problems as creating a drain on self-regulatory strength. Their research suggests that effective self-regulation relies on a "limited and depletable resource." Most of us can only manage so many challenges effectively before they start eroding our ability to regulate demanding behaviors. Managing eating and exercising according to the requirements of a program like the Wellspring Plan certainly creates some demands on our self-regulatory systems. These psychologists' position about strength of self-regulation are summarized: "We labeled this view of self-regulation the 'strength' model, because self-regulation operates like strength: High at first, strength diminishes as the muscles are exerted, and only after some rest is strength restored to its initial power."

Researchers demonstrated these effects in a variety of studies. They had participants attempt to stifle laughter when watching funny films.

Compared to other participants who watched the same films without stifling their natural reactions, those who stifled their emotions initially had greater trouble laughing again when watching subsequent movies.

Weight controllers like Mike, whose situation I described, who deplete their self-regulatory strength, can expect to falter on critical aspects of their weight control programs. What if you could learn ways of managing your emotions so that you could have greater self-regulatory strength? That would allow you to withstand challenges without compromising your program. This chapter intends to show you the way to increase the power of your self-regulatory muscles and to build that strength so that you can become disturbed less by the other aspects of your life. In other words, to help you become *undisturbable*. We will review the nature of stressful situations, describe effective approaches to coping to prepare you to handle such situations more efficiently and also help you understand and begin to use Rational Emotive Therapy (RET) principles. Coping, stress management and RET skills can maximize your self-regulatory strength. In that way, these techniques can help you stay focused and persistent with key weight control behaviors and attitudes.

After reviewing these very helpful and versatile techniques, we will discuss methods of utilizing them to break out of the inevitable slumps that often plague weight controllers: slump busters.

STRESS, STRESSORS AND STRESS MANAGEMENT

Stress and Stressors

Stressors are challenges (demands) from others or from the environment. For some weight controllers, simply passing by a once-favored fast food restaurant can be a stressor. In Mike's situation, he experienced the stressors of his mother's illness and losing his job.

In contrast to stressors, *stress* consists of negative emotional responses to stressors. Stressors can vary in the amount of stress they create for individuals. Overweight young people may experience less stress from the stressor of teasing from cruel classmates if they talk to supportive friends.

Types of Stressors

Stressors create challenges because people struggle to predict or control them. Taunts can come from almost anyone at almost any time. You never know when someone sitting next to you in a meeting or on a train will pull out a candy bar. Much more significant events, such as the death of a family member, separation, divorce or injury, can also be stressors.

Researchers differentiate between two kinds of stressors: "daily hassles" and "major life events." Here are lists which show examples of each type:

Examples of Daily Hassles

- Getting teased
- Failing to find flattering clothes to wear
- Misplacing keys
- Being late
- Performing poorly at a task or a sport
- Failing to understand something
- Worrying about someone else's problems
- Weather problems
- Traffic problems
- Being criticized (recall the stereotype of overweight kids)
- Forgetting something

Examples of Major Life Events

- Changing jobs
- Moving
- Serious illness or injury
- Conflict in a major relationship
- Death of a loved one

It's possible that you may have experienced some discomfort from reading this list as you recall your own reactions to events like these. Would your food choices be affected if you were teased, interrupted from completing something or if you were grappling with a major life event? Would you be able to follow your activity routine according to plan?

STRESS MANAGEMENT TECHNIQUES

Psychologists have studied stress management for decades and know a great deal about those who have the extra strength of self-regulation that enables them to handle stressors without compromising their programs. Sometimes such powerful self-regulators are described as resilient or hardy.

Developing Resilience

Resilient (or hardy) people not only avoid harm from stressors, but they often flourish under this type of pressure. You may recall learning about psychologist Suzanne Kobasa's research on resilience in chapter 2. Dr. Kobasa found that hardy people not only seek to control the challenges they face, as mentioned in chapter 2, but they also rely on two other Cs: commitment and challenge. Those who are committed to their lives and work, who believe they can control their fate and who see stressors as positive challenges, have powerful self-regulatory muscles. They can manage stress quite effectively.

- *Commitment.* Commitment means giving your effort your complete commitment. People with very strong commitments often go through the decision balance sheet procedure described in chapter 6 with very clear advantages for pursuing their goals and with few if any negative consequences for such pursuit. Their programs matter to them a great deal, definitely among the top two to three pursuits in their lives.
- *Control.* Resilient people take charge of the problems they face. They dig in, find out how to solve them or determine the approach most likely to produce benefits.
- *Challenge.* Resilient weight controllers don't let setbacks or disappointments derail them. Successful weight controllers don't stop looking at scales or looking at mirrors. They keep moving forward, committing to making a positive change in their lives and to looking at the many aspects of successful weight control as challenges, not stressors.

To become more resilient yourself, consider responding to stressors by asking questions that direct you to take charge. Ask yourself:

- What can I do to eliminate this stressor?
- How can I look at this problem as an opportunity for change and growth?
- In what ways does this stressor teach me something about my life?
- How can I use this situation to improve my functioning or competence?

Try adding these questions to your personal lexicon at home. Talk in terms of challenges and opportunities rather than talking about problems in whiny and hopeless tones. In plain terms, it's making lemonade (sugar-free, of course) out of lemons.

Stress Inoculation

University of Waterloo psychologist Don Meichenbaum developed a useful approach for handling major stressors. Called stress inoculation, this technique builds "psychological antibodies" by preventing the attachment of problematic emotions like anger and anxiety to stressors. Stress inoculation includes an educational phase and a coping self-talk phase.

- *Education about the Stressor.* In this phase of stress inoculation, fear of the unknown is abated with important information about the stressor. For example, children going to the dentist for the first time may not know what happens there. A friend may have told them that it hurts or that a big person in a white coat will yank out their teeth with a pair of pliers. When facing a stressor, it's generally beneficial to try to understand, read about and take other steps to educate yourself about it.
- *Coping Self-Statements.* We all talk to ourselves, at least sometimes. You may have done so when you first dove off a diving board or made your first public speech. Perhaps you made self-statements like "C'mon, you can do it," or "Go for it." Research shows that such self-statements are actually quite helpful when facing challenges of all kinds. Psychologists advise people facing such challenges to use four types of self-statements: preparing for the stressor, confronting and handling the stressor, coping with feelings at critical moments and rewarding oneself for successful coping.

Here are examples of these four types of self-statements that can be used to manage almost any stressor. By using these self-statements, you can begin to cope with stressors more actively and become more resilient.

Self-Statements when Preparing for a Stressor
- What do I have to do?
- I can create a plan to deal with this.

- Thinking about what I have to do is certainly better than getting nervous about it.
- Worrying won't help. Plan.
- My anxiety tells me that I have a challenge facing me.
- I can learn from this.
- Remain logical and calm.

Self-Statements when Confronting and Handling the Stressor
- I can handle this.
- I can meet this challenge.
- Just take it one step at a time; follow the plan.
- Beat the fear: think of what I am doing.
- Relax. I'm in control. Just take a slow, deep breath.
- My tension just tells me to follow my plan; deal with this challenge.
- I can eat safe foods as part of my plan.

Self-Statements when Coping with Feelings at Critical Moments
- When tension comes, just pause and breathe slowly.
- Focus on the present. Now, what do I have to do?
- I've handled this before and I can manage it now.
- I'll rate my fear from one to ten and then watch it change.
- I'll just keep the tension manageable; I won't worry about eliminating it altogether.
- I can do this. It will be over in a certain amount of time.
- Okay, keep focused on what I want to do.
- This is not the worst thing that can happen.
- Remember, I don't have to handle this perfectly, just reasonably well.
- Focus on sensations: coldness, warmth, smells, touch, taste, sights and sounds.
- Think about other times and places. Good feelings come with good thoughts.
- I'm in control.
- If I'm going to overeat, I'll deviate quantitatively, not qualitatively.

Self-Statements when Rewarding Oneself for Successful Coping
- Nice going! I was able to do it.
- It wasn't as tough as I expected.
- Wait 'til I tell [a friend, a family member] about it.
- I'm making progress.
- My plan worked.
- I'm learning all the time.
- It's my thinking that creates anxiety. When I control my self-statements, I can control my anxiety.
- I'm doing better each time I use these self-statements.
- I'm really pleased with my progress.

Weight controllers face many stressors that can directly impact weight control. Consider a typical holiday party. These holiday parties usually include lots of high-fat foods and a generally relaxed and unrestrained state. How could you use the stress inoculation approach to handle this stressor?

First, you would learn as much as possible about the event:

- How many people will be there?
- What kind of food will be served?
- More specifically, are there options for the main course and are there good (very low-fat) options during the hors d'oeuvres or early phases of the party?
- Will there be friends I'll enjoy talking with or will I be bored?
- Will I be able to leave when I feel like it?

The answers to these questions determine the severity of the stressor. The party can be easily managed if low-fat options abound and if socializing provides a good distraction. On the other hand, a boring party combined with abundant high-fat food may require a higher level of coping skills.

Coping self-statements can help get you through challenges like this. Try some of the following:

Preparing

- I can create a plan that will get me through this.
- I don't have to worry about this; I can plan for it.

- I'm sure I can learn from this and get even better at managing these kinds of situations.
- Plan:
    1. Get a diet cola or a sparkling water and hang on to it.
    2. Find the most interesting people available and talk with them.
    3. Convince the person I came with to leave if I give him/her the signal.

Confronting and Handling

- I can handle this.
- There are a lot of people here, but that gives me greater choices.
- Stay focused and remember that everything counts.

Coping at Critical Moments

- If I see some tempting morsel in the hors d'oeuvre phase, I'll grip my diet drink even more tightly.
- Remember to find some low-fat alternatives; they've got to be here.
- Even if I eat some problematic foods, I can still count it and record it.
- Every food has finite calories and fat grams; nothing is going to kill me here.
- Let me find somebody I can talk to who can make me laugh.
- Even if the main course is high in fat, I don't have to eat a lot of it.

Rewarding Myself for Success

- Nice going. I basically followed the plan.
- The plan was good even though I did eat a few things I didn't want to.
- I think I'm getting better at this.

Cued Relaxation. Cued relaxation is a way of including relaxation in everyday life by using cues to remind yourself to take a brief relaxation break. Such cues can include a ringing cell phone, drinking water, reaching for a wallet, brushing hair or applying makeup. When the cue occurs, take a few seconds to use a relaxation technique.

Here are a few examples.

Cue = Ringing cell phone

1. Cell phone rings.
2. Answer phone.
3. Use a breathing technique (e.g., slow rhythmic breathing).
4. During the call, focus on breathing in a relaxed manner.
5. After the call, take another few seconds to execute the relaxation technique once again.

Cue = Drinking Water or Diet Soda

1. Begin drinking.
2. Focus on the liquid and the sounds and sights of it.
   - What color is it?
   - What specifically does it sound like as you drink?
   - Concentrate on the texture of the fluid as it enters your mouth and goes down your throat.
3. Create a vivid image that involves water:
   - You are on a beach in the summertime and you are watching a wave gently flow to the shore and retreat.
   - You are hiking on a mountain and you come upon a beautiful waterfall. You are watching the water flow and beat down on the rocks below. You are listening to the sounds and smelling the air.
4. Take a few minutes to stay in the image, keeping it vivid, using all of your senses to enliven the imagery.

Cue = Reaching for Your Wallet

1. After your hand makes contact with the wallet, remind yourself to relax.
2. Tense and then relax some of the muscles in your hand and arm. Tense and relax those muscles at least twice.

3. Pay attention to the change in sensation from the tense to the relaxed state for each muscle group that you use. Focus on the relaxed state for a few seconds and try to bring that sense of relaxation from the top of your head through your eyes and down to the rest of your body.

When You Use Food to Cope. When food is used as a coping response to a stressor, you can deviate quantitatively, not qualitatively. This means consuming very low-fat foods when stressed, even large quantities of them, but avoiding high-fat foods altogether.

This approach works better because it keeps the goal of very low-fat eating clearly in mind at all times. If weight controllers occasionally eat higher-fat foods in response to stress, then they no longer use the very low-fat standard consistently. Clearer goals produce better outcomes than fuzzier goals. This means that once you begin enjoying very low-fat foods, it's much easier to continue the progress if you deviate quantitatively in response to stressors (for example, eating several servings of fat-free chocolate pudding) rather than qualitatively (for example, eating several slices of pizza with regular-fat cheese). So, just remember this suggestion and you will take an important step toward long-term success:

Deviate quantitatively, not qualitatively.

This concept is sufficiently important to consider typing it in a large, bold font and putting it on your fridge (along with the calendar you're using to track steps).

Five Steps to Keep Lapses from Becoming Relapses

LAPSE ≠ RELAPSE

Biology and our obesogenic environment make it impossible for anyone to eat perfectly. You will do better, especially in the long run, if you accept the fact you can't achieve perfection in eating. Lapses are inevitable. It's important not to view a lapse as a tragedy. A lapse is a temporary problem, a temporary detour from the overall plan. A lapse does not have to lead to relapse, which is defined as a full-blown change back into old problematic patterns of eating and inactivity.

In our Wellspring programs, our participants learn a particular five-step road map to managing lapses in a way that seems to prevent them from becoming relapses. It includes these five steps:

1. **Acceptance.** It happened. No one died. Overeating in any form is not a major criminal offense. It's just a problematic behavior. Masterful weight control does not require perfection. It's a tough taskmaster with biological and social-environmental challenges every single day.

2. **Hit the Replay Button.** Replay what happened in your mind's eye. Take into account your personal situation at the moment of the lapse (e.g., perhaps you had not eaten anything for many hours or were very distracted by something in your life). Then, analyze the situation (e.g., party; eating in a high-risk situation; other people's behaviors).

3. **Replay it with Corrective Action.** Imagine what you could have done to avoid the problematic eating. For example, what if you ate some French fries offered to you by a friend at a fast food restaurant? Corrective action could include saying "No thanks" or eating a salad instead. It could also include suggesting an alternative place to eat. Just play out a good alternative in your imagination.

4. **Self-monitor.** Record the specifics of what you ate, calories and fat grams.

5. **Move On.** Some people think it helps to exercise more on a day with a lapse or eat less following the lapse. This type of punishment can easily backfire. You can find the corrective measures of this sort so onerous that you might skip steps one to four the next time you lapse. Skipping those steps could lead to discontinuing your weight control efforts altogether, throwing out the baby with the bath water. By simply moving on with your day, you acknowledge the difficulty of the task itself appropriately. Weight control demands a great deal from you. It does not demand perfection. When slip-ups occur, merely acknowledging them, accepting them and figuring out how best to avoid them in the next situation like the one you faced will serve you best.

Top Ten High-Risk Situations and How to Cope with Them

Take a few minutes to complete the survey of high-risk situations in Exercise 11-1.

Exercise 11-1: High-Risk Situations

Please rank the following situations based on how difficult they are for you to manage and stay on program (i.e., maintaining very low-fat eating). Rank **only** the five most challenging situations in order of how hard they are for you. The hardest should be almost impossible. The 5th should still be quite challenging.

_____ Right after arriving home from school or work
_____ Watching TV in the evening
_____ Watching a movie in a theater
_____ Attending a sporting event
_____ Studying
_____ Reading
_____ Using a computer
_____ Eating in a restaurant with friends
_____ Eating in a restaurant with family
_____ Attending a party
_____ Eating a holiday meal
_____ Eating at a friend's or a relative's house
_____ Eating lunch at school or work
_____ Feeling bored
_____ Feeling depressed or anxious
_____ Feeling happy or relaxed
_____ Feeling hungry
_____ Having a craving
_____ After eating a particularly unsatisfying meal
_____ Feeling tired
_____ Shopping alone
_____ Shopping with others
_____ Eating dinner with my family at home
_____ Other (please specify): _____

More than one hundred Wellspring participants rated the following ten situations as the most challenging. Let's consider each of these high-risk situations and review some potentially useful coping responses that Wellspring participants have found quite helpful.

#1: Eating in a Restaurant with Friends

At [the diner], we utilize whatever bit of autonomy we have to ply our customers with the illicit calories that signal our love. It is our job as servers to assemble the salads and desserts, pour the dressings and squirt the whipped cream. We also control the number of butter pats our customers get and the amount of sour cream on their baked potatoes. So if you wonder why Americans are so obese, consider the fact that waitresses both express their humanity and earn their tips through the covert distribution of fats.

—*Barbara Ehrenreich*, <u>Nickel and Dimed in America</u>

As described in chapter 3, we're eating out much more often—nearly twice as frequently as we did a generation ago. When we eat out, we are giving up control over ingredients, method of preparation and portion size. We also don't control the atmosphere, which often can lull you into making problematic food choices. To counteract those forces, it takes some preparation and an appropriate orientation to the challenges at hand.

Try remembering these points:

- It is your right to request that the food you order at a restaurant be prepared according to your wishes—your right to get what you pay for.
- Most restaurateurs want to accommodate their patrons. In a recent survey conducted by a major credit card company, more than 90 percent of restaurateurs said they preferred hearing complaints about orders directly. They want you to be satisfied and come back again and again.
- Still, some servers resist providing you with the information you want about food preparation. Remind yourself of your right to this information. Then, try making a polite request, even repeated requests, if necessary.

This approach will work well most of the time. Here's an interaction that illustrates how to make it work:

> ***Patron:*** *I'll take the chicken with broccoli and new potatoes. How is that prepared?*
>
> ***Server:*** *How is what prepared?*
>
> ***Patron:*** *The chicken.*
>
> ***Server:*** *I think it's broiled.*
>
> ***Patron:*** *In other words, it might be sautéed instead of broiled?*
>
> ***Server:*** *Yeah.*
>
> ***Patron:*** *Could you check on that for me, please?*
>
> ***Server:*** *I will.*
>
> *(Server leaves for two minutes to check on preparation of the chicken and then returns.)*
>
> ***Server:*** *It's broiled.*
>
> ***Patron:*** *Great. Then I'll go with the chicken. I'd like the vegetables grilled, with no butter added on them.*
>
> ***Server:*** *I don't think they put any butter on the vegetables or the potatoes.*
>
> ***Patron:*** *Please check that no butter or any sauces are added to the broccoli or the potatoes.*
>
> ***Server:*** *Okay.*

Does this patron seem overly pushy to you? If you answered yes, you will likely have a problem managing this highest risk situation. Getting what you pay for includes knowing what you're getting. If your server does not comply with reasonable requests for this kind of information, you could ask to speak to the manager or the owner. You could also leave the restaurant. Remaining at a restaurant and eating foods you want to avoid simply does not work for weight controllers.

Wellspring participants sometimes lament the limited choices in certain types of restaurants which serve ethnic foods. Another very challenging restaurant: small-town diners.

Table 11-1 presents a list of challenging cuisines and some suggestions from Wellspring alumni.

Table 11-1
Challenging Cuisines—Suggestions for Very Low-Fat Meals

- **Cajun:** Seafood or vegetable gumbo or jambalaya (without sausage), grilled fish
- **Chinese:** First, ask what can be prepared without oil. Stir-fries prepared with fat-free sauces, broths or soy sauce; chicken, seafood and vegetables; soups (hot and sour, chicken, vegetable); chicken and shrimp dishes steamed without sauces
- **Diners:** Chicken dinner (grilled or broiled) with baked potato and mixed vegetables (steamed); if there's a vegetarian special, order it prepared without butter or oil.
- **French:** Poached, grilled or steamed fish; chicken and wine sauce; Niçoise salads without oil
- **Greek:** Chicken and fish shish kebabs; salads, couscous, rice
- **Indian:** Tandoori chicken, prawns, fish
- **Italian:** Pasta with red clam sauce, meatless marinara without oil; pizza with no cheese and steamed vegetable toppings; minestrone soup (made without butter)
- **Japanese:** Sushi, chicken and fish teriyaki, tofu and vegetables (avoid avocado, mayonnaise, eel and mackerel)
- **Mexican:** Chicken and seafood enchiladas with no cheese or sour cream; tamales with no cheese, chicken or shrimp fajitas (without sour cream, guacamole) and made with "as little oil as possible;" chicken taco salad (no cheese); salsa (request tortillas as a side dish to dip into salsa instead of chips)
- **Thai:** First, ask what can be prepared without oil. Then, stir-fried shrimp, chicken and vegetable dishes can work for you. Also, soups, especially sweet and sour (Tom Yum) soup; chicken and cucumber salads

A critical saying to remember when ordering in restaurants is:

If you don't know what the food is or how it was prepared, assume the worst!

This saying directs you to find something on the menu you can rely on. If you look diligently enough, you too "can always find something to eat," no matter how challenging the menu.

#2: Eating at a Friend's or Relative's House, #3: Eating a Holiday Meal and #4: Attending a Party

We address all these issues in this section, because the effective coping responses are similar. These high-risk situations tend to invoke a free-spirit, "just have fun" attitude. Although these events are enjoyable, they do challenge the focus and consistency necessary for effective weight control. But by using effective strategies, all of these stressors can be managed.

Consider Thanksgiving, a holiday that most Americans consider a day for a well-justified eating frenzy and probably the extreme example of this category of high-risk situations. Here's a fairly typical Thanksgiving meal:

Foods/Serving Size	Calories
Turkey (no skin, one-half white, one-half dark meat) - 3 oz	148
Mashed potatoes - 1 cup	222
Gravy—½ cup	61
Stuffing—½ cup	250
Candied sweet potato - 1	144
Cranberry sauce - 2 Tablespoons	52
Fresh fruit salad—½ cup	62
Celery - 1 stalk	5
Carrots—½ cup	15
Bread - 1 roll	71
Butter - 1 pat	35
Pumpkin pie - 2 slices	600
Whipped cream—¼ cup	200
Coffee	0
Total	**1,865**

This meal more than doubles the calorie-conscious limit of 800 calories at the biggest meal of the day. But many of these menu items pose no major problems: white meat turkey without the skin, potatoes, fresh fruit salad, celery and carrots. It's the stuffing, gravy, butter, pumpkin pie crust and whipped cream that pile on the fat and calories. By selecting the low-fat components of the classic Thanksgiving dinner, you can have an excellent meal and a wonderful time.

The Christmas season poses even greater risks for weight controllers. Unlike Thanksgiving, Easter and parties at friends' houses, Christmas festivities last well beyond one particular day. Many people attend pre-Christmas parties and mini-celebrations. We often find ourselves surrounded by sugary treats at schools, offices and in many homes. Many families enjoy rituals involving Christmas cookies and the like—all during a time of year when the weather can make staying active especially challenging.

Weight controllers use several tricks of the trade during the holidays. These strategies apply equally well to eating at a friend's house or attending a birthday party. Consider the following suggestions for the holiday season:

Plan Ahead

When you plan ahead, you can predict and control your world. Think about the next birthday party you'll attend. Who's going to be there and what kind of food will be served? Call the host and get a preview of the menu. You can make a tentative list of what you'll eat, who you'll talk to and how to stay focused.

Self-monitor

It is particularly important to self-monitor during the holiday season. As routines change, consistency of self-monitoring often decreases. This compounds the challenges. Also, when you're at other people's homes and at parties, your ability to identify cooking methods and ingredients is diminished. Try to come up with a bottom-line estimate of the number of fat grams consumed every day, even if the accuracy may not be great. The focus required for such estimates keeps weight controllers connected to their long-term goals and nurtures the healthy obsession.

Avoid Starvation before Celebration

Starving before a big holiday meal can produce binge eating. Starving produces deprivation and a very strong biological response to the sight of food. This biological response includes the secretion of insulin and saliva. If you eat nothing or very little before a big holiday meal or party, you will get incredibly hungry and are more likely to make bad decisions. A better approach is to enjoy low-fat, low-sugar foods for breakfast and lunch. Having a small snack just before leaving for the party may help as well.

Scope Out the Food Scene

After arriving at the location for the party, you can quickly survey the available options. Perhaps there are fresh vegetables and other healthy snacks that will work for you. You may also learn that the main course is a low-fat chicken, pasta or fish dish. This knowledge may be the key to provide you with the control you need to keep away from the high-fat snacks.

Use a Food Plan

Once you are aware of what's available, you can develop a specific food plan for what you'll eat and a way of focusing on that plan. For example, you can hold a glass of diet cola or water and focus attention on the conversation instead of the food. You can also use this cue or some other cue (perhaps munching vegetables) to remind yourself of your immediate and long-range goals. Write out this plan in advance and then see how your self-monitoring records match up immediately afterwards.

Refocus Your Holiday Season

This suggestion goes well beyond an individual event or party. Holidays are traditionally focused around food and celebrations. You can break this tradition by focusing on other people or special projects and finding new, creative ways to relax. You might develop some skills in winter sports (ice skating, skiing), focus on enjoying board games in front of a crackling fire or reading good books.

#5: Right After Arriving Home from School or Work, #6: Feeling Bored, #7: Feeling Depressed or Anxious and #8: Using a Computer

All four of these high-risk situations involve limited movement and common emotional states. If you can learn to use activity to manage emotions and reduce sedentary activity more generally, the entire process gets a lot easier.

Movement Helps

Maintaining a high activity level helps weight controllers in many ways, including reducing appetite and improving mood. When you think of the billions of dollars spent on medications that reduce appetite and improve mood, it's amazing to recognize that studies have shown that even ten minutes of brisk walking produces significant improvements in mood, for free!

Although we reviewed this research in the chapter on food, it's worth taking another look. Robert Thayer, a psychologist at California State University, compared the results of eating a small candy bar (½ oz) versus taking a ten-minute brisk walk. As shown in the next figure, walking led to more energy and lower tension, whereas the candy bar had the opposite effect.

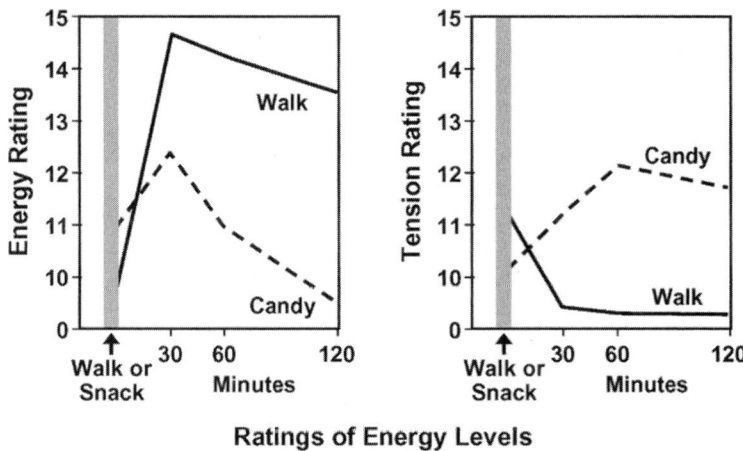

Ratings of Energy Levels

Cheryl Hansen and her colleagues from Northern Arizona University wanted to see if ten, twenty or thirty minutes of exercise produced different degrees of improvements in mood. The researchers monitored what happened when their twenty-one college students rode exercise bikes at a fairly comfortable, but somewhat strenuous intensity: 60 percent of maximum aerobic capacity. They found that even just ten minutes on the bike produced substantial improvements in mood.

These improvements in mood send a message worth memorizing:

> *When the going gets rough, get going—
> even if just for ten minutes.*

#9: Feeling Hungry and #10: Having a Craving

Most diets focus on hunger and cravings as if they account for 98 percent of problems in weight control. The biology of excess weight makes hunger quite complex. Let's define hunger very simply: the desire for food. What do you think causes you to get hungry? Take a look at the factors in Table 11-2 to see the wide range of variables that affect judgments about hunger.

Table 11-2
Hungry?

Here are some factors influencing the intensity of hunger:

- Biology (e.g., fat cells)
- Eating by others (e.g., parties)
- Consumption of alcohol, marijuana and other recreational drugs
- Emotions (e.g., stress, anger, frustration, boredom, etc.)
- Activities (e.g., exercise; amount of activity)
- Fat consumption
- Fiber
- Negative thoughts (e.g., "I've blown it already today.")
- Presence of foods, particularly highly appealing foods
- Protein consumption
- Stimuli that are associated with eating (e.g., in the car, TV)
- Sugar consumption
- Talking about food
- Thinking about food
- Time of day and normal routines
- Tiredness
- Variety/blandness of diet
- Volume of food

This list of eighteen factors helps make the case that you cannot rely on some notion of hunger to impact what you eat, if you want to succeed as a weight controller. Those excess fat cells and associated hormones and enzymes would like you to eat constantly, especially after you lost weight. Instead, you must rely on the factors in the food chapter (chapter 7) to quiet your desire for food and achieve your goals. Your goals establish a limit on fat consumption per day and calories per meal.

You can also understand cravings and learn to manage them. Cravings are a very strong desire for food (perhaps stimulated by biological forces associated with weight loss or by not eating for a while) coupled with an idea. The idea could include a particular food or image of some food (like pizza or chocolate). The best antidotes for cravings are:

- Distraction: Focus on other things, make a phone call or send a text or e-mail.
- Activity: Even a ten minute walk, as noted earlier
- Eating: Something safe (but lovable)

EIGHT ADDITIONAL SLUMP MAKERS OR CHALLENGES

In addition to the challenges posed in the preceding sections, like lapses and eating at restaurants, here are eight others that can threaten this new lifestyle you've developed. Understanding these challenges may help you anticipate and manage them more effectively.

Injuries and Illnesses

Momentum is a magical thing. In weight control, you can build momentum for change. You can get into routines and rely on those routines to keep you going. Those routines are the lifeblood of your healthy obsession. Twisted ankles, bad backs, flus, colds and other problems can impede your momentum by changing your routines.

Poorly managed injuries and illnesses can kill momentum for effective weight control. For example, one of my clients, David, developed chronic sinus infections after the birth of his second child. Children bring a lot of joy into life—but a lot of colds as well. David had allergy problems, but his children's "gift" of frequent colds increased his problems. Sinus infections are like mild colds that also produce fevers and sluggishness. Unfortunately, they don't go away in seven days. They tend to stick around for weeks or months, if untreated by antibiotics. David found it difficult to maintain his jogging program, and thereby control his weight, because of these sinus infections.

He went to see an ear, nose and throat specialist and an allergist. After a variety of tests, David's doctors decided the best course of action for him was to use very strong doses of antibiotics and also to "take it easier, listen to your body and don't exercise so much."

Weight controllers also experience injuries. As you become more active in managing your program, even by increasing your steps consistently, overuse injuries will occur occasionally. Your back could become strained or you could develop knee, hip or foot problems. These momentum busters pose very real challenges. Athletes push their bodies hard. Successful weight controllers push their bodies hard as well.

Scale Phobia

"I didn't want to get on a scale this week because I think I gained weight." Does this sound familiar? It's a problematic attitude that can lead to lapses and slumps. Scales provide critical information to weight controllers that can assist in setting goals and changing patterns associated with weight gain. Recent research suggests the benefits of weighing yourself every day. If you get into that habit, then your healthy obsession will get stronger.

Vacations

Most people find vacations relaxing, distracting and enjoyable. Vacations are also dangerous to weight controllers. Vacations interfere with momentum. Vacations, like illnesses and injuries, cause changes in your usual routines. One of my clients, Renee, said, "I get into a 'vacation mentality.' The vacation mentality gets me to relax my restraint. I take it easy on myself. I don't force myself to exercise or count calories. I focus on my family and have fun." You can see that a "vacation mentality" can become a dangerous thing. Vacations can lead to decreases in exercise and re-emergence of higher-fat, higher-sugar eating. Once these patterns reemerge, they become hard to kill off again.

Changes in Key Relationships

Major conflicts in key relationships can interfere with your life more dramatically than almost anything else. What happened to you the last time you had a major conflict at work? Most people report trouble sleeping and tremendous preoccupation when such conflicts occur. Conflicts at home produce even more dramatic symptoms. Major lapses can quickly become slumps during periods of conflict with friends, co-workers and loved ones. The sense of "nothing else matters" can sap your self-regulation strength, making effective eating and exercising seem absolutely trivial during these difficult times.

Work or Financial Crises

Losing a job or suffering major financial problems can interfere substantially with weight control. These crises, like crises in personal relationships, can make weight control seem unimportant by comparison.

I've heard many clients say, "How can I worry about the number of fat grams I eat when my world is crumbling around me?" Considerable self-regulatory resources must now be diverted into consolidating resources, networking and re-thinking careers.

Major Changes in Eating Environments

The following two stories show how major changes in environments can affect your eating patterns dramatically.

> *Arnie*: "I got promoted a few months ago. I was really excited. It was a great opportunity. Unfortunately, it involved traveling two to three days per week. I figured, 'No big deal, I can handle this.' I didn't realize how much traveling around the country disrupted my usual routines. I found myself frustrated and irritated more of the time. Relaxation and cooling down time became less and less. I felt tired in the morning and found it difficult to exercise at my usual time. I wound up in meetings in which all kinds of food (like muffins, doughnuts, pizza, cheese and crackers) were carted in during all hours of the day and night. My eating and exercising habits began to break down, and I began gaining weight."
>
> *Jane*: "I got a divorce last year. The time before the divorce was the real struggle (for about two years). The divorce was a tremendous relief for me. My weight was reasonably stable during the years before the divorce. I couldn't believe it, but I gained twenty pounds during this past year. It was such an adjustment. All of a sudden, for the first time in ten years, I was living by myself. I thought that would make it so much easier to control my food. I didn't realize that being in an unhappy relationship in some ways created fewer temptations for me than being alone. I found myself feeling lonely. Other times, I went out with friends to dinners and parties—far more often than I had in the last ten years. I was drinking more and eating bar food. I had more trouble sleeping, and that made it harder to get up early and exercise. I guess that's what did it."

As discussed in earlier chapters, traveling creates many challenges for weight controllers. Any substantial modification in your living situation also creates problems to be solved. Moving out of your house and into a college dormitory, or moving out of a dormitory into an apartment, are transitions with which you are probably familiar. If you recall those transitions in your life, consider the impact they had on your eating and exercising. Have you ever heard of the "Freshman Fifteen?" Many college freshmen report gaining fifteen pounds when they move into a college dormitory for the first time. These weight gains, while not documented scientifically, may occur for some people because of the tremendous changes in their usual routines.

Poor Problem Solving

A recent study compared "maintainers" to "re-gainers." Maintainers were formerly overweight women who had lost at least twenty pounds and maintained that loss for at least two years. Re-gainers were overweight women who regained weight after losing at least twenty pounds. Re-gainers used "escape-avoidance" methods of solving problems much more so than did maintainers. These methods included eating, drinking, smoking, sleeping and wishing the problems would just go away. Re-gainers also failed to get as much support from others ("social support") as did the maintainers.

Abstinence Violation Effect

Psychologists have identified a type of distortion in thinking that creates problems. The abstinence violation effect, or AVE, first involves making a commitment to "abstinence." Many people who change their habits (for example, people who quit smoking or stop drinking alcohol, as well as successful weight controllers) make a commitment to abstain forever from a certain pattern of eating or drinking. Weight controllers who do this may view themselves as "dieters."

What happens when a dieter eats a food that is not on the diet? For example, what happens when someone on a low-carb diet eats a piece of birthday cake? This dieter may view this initial lapse as a major conflict. The conflict might sound something like this in the mind of the dieter: "How can I be a dieter if I ate a piece of birthday cake?" One way of resolving this conflict is to abandon dieting. In other words, abstinence violation effects can be relapses that occur to reduce the internal conflict created by lapses. When weight controllers commit to unrealistically stringent standards for eating or exercising, they set the stage for AVEs. Following this type of unrealistic commitment, initial lapses can produce serious conflicts. These internal conflicts can then be resolved by launching a full-blown slump, "I can eat cake now because I'm no longer a dieter." If you view yourself instead as a weight controller committed to permanent lifestyle change, then you will prevent such extreme reactions to minor lapses.

SLUMP-BUSTERS

Whether your slump was caused by an injury, scale phobia, a vacation, stinkin' thinkin' or something else, now what? The following suggestions require action! Insight alone won't do it. Regaining momentum requires some notable action that leads to an even more notable change in your life.

Re-visit Your Healthy Obsession

When consistent exercisers stop exercising, even for one day, they get rather testy. When weight controllers find their usual routines of eating, exercising and monitoring disrupted, they also get testy. These individuals rely on a certain approach to eating and exercising and observing themselves in order to feel comfortable. Disruptions become sources of annoyance, irritability and dissatisfaction. This is the heart of a healthy obsession, defining successful weight controllers; it shows a very strong commitment to permanent weight control.

Some weight controllers become secretly happy when opportunities to stray from their usual patterns emerge. You may have noticed this in yourself or others. "Oh well, I was at a party and there was nothing else to eat—so I ate!" If you truly embrace a healthy obsession, you will hold yourself to a higher standard. You would find it unacceptable to deviate from your plans without dealing with those deviations as problems. This doesn't mean that you berate yourself unmercifully when problems develop. It does mean that you see deviations as problems and attempt to deal with them directly. Wouldn't it be great if successful weight control meant having a happy-go-lucky attitude and feeling free of the oppression that seems required for success? It just doesn't work that way. The biology of excess weight is simply too tenacious. It takes a certain level of control, focusing and intensity to manage it effectively.

Some of my clients who have lost a lot of weight and kept it off for years have lamented, "Now that I've lost all this weight, I expected to feel good about myself most of the time. But I don't. I still struggle with my eating habits every day." Sadly, this is the nature of the battle with the biology of excess weight. Most people do not view their own successes at weight control as joyous accomplishments. People who lose a lot of weight are typically less than thrilled about their new weight statuses. Usually, they want to lose another five, ten, twenty or more pounds. Even if they find their new weights acceptable, they still have to work hard to maintain their focus. There may be a certain "joy in the discipline." Exercise can bring its own rewards, as can a sense of control about eating patterns. Nevertheless, the state in which many successful weight controllers find themselves feels more like "healthy obsession" than "joyous accomplishment."

Health Clubs

Many years ago, health clubs were places for fanatics, weightlifters, grunters and athletes. Now, they serve as social melting pots. They also provide many comforts and a wide range of activities. Low-impact and no-impact aerobic classes, spinning classes, water aerobics activities, yoga, instruction in almost every indoor sport imaginable and machines, machines, machines. These centers of physical activity can serve as effective slump-busters. When people join such centers, they tend to use them, at least for a while. Their novelty and diversity of activities can motivate refocusing on healthy eating and exercising.

When selecting a health club, keep in mind their three most important qualities: location, location, location! You will find that you actually use your health club when you either live very near it or work near it. If you belong to a health club located close to your house, you may use it in the morning. Almost all of the thousands of weight controllers with whom I have worked over the last forty years, and who have succeeded at this difficult enterprise, have exercised primarily in the morning. Morning exercise proves most reliable because it interferes less in your daily life. After all, in the morning, you have complete control of your schedule and you can exercise before getting showered and dressed for the day. Exercising at any other time of the day could require taking a second shower and interrupting activities. Yet another advantage of morning exercise concerns attitude. You may have noticed that you feel better during the day if you exercise first thing in the morning. For all of these reasons, consider choosing a health club near your home if at all possible.

Personal Trainers

Many people use trainers to help motivate them. Working with a trainer can help you learn about different types of equipment. For example, if you decide to begin a weightlifting program, a trainer could provide important instruction on technique and help you set up an effective regimen. Trainers can also provide encouragement and support. If you set up an appointment with a trainer, and particularly if you prepay for that appointment, you will motivate yourself, increasing your chances of doing some constructive exercising that day.

Try to find trainers who have advanced degrees in physical education or who are certified as athletic trainers. The American College of Sports Medicine certifies trainers. The world's largest group that certifies trainers is the American Council on Exercise (ACE). ACE Certified Trainers have passed a rigorous test demonstrating a detailed knowledge of physical exercise and conditioning principles. If you select a trainer who has an advanced degree in physical education and/or appropriate certification, you can feel more confident that the advice you get is grounded in science rather than hearsay. Unfortunately, personal trainers can cost from ten to one hundred dollars per hour. Prices vary depending on the standards used within the health club, training and whether the trainers come to your house or you go to their facilities. If you are in a major slump, paying the price of weekly sessions with a personal trainer for a month or two may be helpful.

Equipment

"I couldn't get myself focused until I bought a treadmill. It was a major expense (almost $2000), but I get on that thing every day now. I really like it. I like having it in my house because of the flexibility and the reminder it provides. When I see it sitting there (which is very easy because it's huge), I know how important my program is to me." These sentiments were expressed by one of my former clients. She had indeed gotten into a major slump and was very excited about the way her new treadmill helped her get out of it.

An equipment purchase can prove very motivating for the reasons this former client outlined. Having the equipment in your home makes it much easier to exercise. Many people who have weight problems are reluctant to go to health clubs. They find the looks and comments of other people disconcerting. Of course, overweight people have as much right to use facilities at health clubs as anyone else. Yet, the feelings can be so strong for some people that overcoming them is very difficult. Some people also live in climates that make outdoor exercising, such as walking or jogging, particularly challenging. These challenges can be overcome with appropriate clothing. However, when it's ten degrees below or icy, you won't find even hardy souls merrily walking around outside.

Some very adequate exercycles are available for a few hundred dollars. More elaborate pieces of quality equipment carry much higher price tags. The best way to decide which piece of equipment makes the most sense for you is to go to a health club and try out the equipment. If you try out various types of equipment for several weeks, you will determine which kind is most comfortable for you and which you might use consistently.

Consumer Reports routinely evaluates exercise equipment for home use. Your local library usually has copies of recent issues of *Consumer Reports* and you can get an online subscription for electronic devices. The publisher of this magazine also prints books and maintains a convenient website that summarizes their findings. Before spending hundreds of dollars, perhaps thousands, consider studying the available evidence about which pieces of equipment work most effectively and reliably.

Radical Changes in Diet

Radical changes in eating plans can sometimes break slumps. They require concentration, but may serve as rallying points for change. Usually, radical dietary approaches suffer the same fate as all diets: They do not work for very long. But as a temporary step, making a major shift in your eating plan could spark important changes. You could try, for example, a vegetarian approach.

Medications

Joe, an obviously overweight middle-aged man, went to see his doctor about the new "diet" medications.

> *Joe*: Doc, I've got to have those new meds that will get me to believe I just ate a turkey dinner.
>
> *Doctor*: Well, Joe, I don't know about the turkey dinner part, but they could help you lose weight if you're willing to work at it.
>
> *Joe*: But Doc, I thought those pills made you feel like you just ate a turkey dinner and then they also make you really want to work at it.
>
> *Doctor*: Sorry Joe. To really want to work at it, you have to find that within yourself somewhere—not in your medicine cabinet.

Physicians began prescribing amphetamines more than fifty years ago to help people lose weight. Unfortunately, not only do amphetamines reduce appetite, they are addictive drugs that produce a "high" that people crave. Thousands of people became addicted to amphetamines in an attempt to lose weight. These drugs can no longer be prescribed in the United States or England for weight control. Prescriptions for these medications are carefully monitored by governmental agencies.

Many physicians know this sad tale. They believe that any drug prescribed for weight control may cause more harm than good. They may well be right about this. For example, one of the few medications for weight loss with current FDA approval contains an enzyme that blocks the absorption of fat, at least the absorption of about one-third of the fat consumed. Some preliminary research suggests that at least some people respond favorably to taking this medication and lose modest amounts of weight. However, if you follow the principles in this book (for example, eating as little fat as possible), the drug would not prove helpful. In addition, most people will experience some notable and troublesome digestive problems associated with taking a medication that extracts fat from food (including flatulence, oily stools and bloating).

Successful weight controllers tend to find ways to eat low-fat foods and make that a permanent part of their lifestyles. Reliance on this medication for that purpose seems unlikely as an effective long-term strategy. On the other hand, you could occasionally use a medication like this if you do overeat high-fat foods. If taken within an hour of the problematic food or meal, it could decrease the impact of eating high-fat foods.

It is critical to emphasize that it only makes sense to take these medications if you are participating in a professionally conducted weight control program. Scientific research suggests that these medications produce few benefits unless weight controllers get help focusing on eating and exercising through a professional program while they are taking them.

If prescription medications for weight control can help some participants in professional programs, can over-the-counter drugs help anyone? Probably not. One of the two non-prescription drugs that are available in the United States, phenylpropanolamine (PPA), acts like a mild stimulant. PPA can produce some small weight losses, but the effects do not last long. PPA is found in most non-prescription "weight control" drugs. Benzocaine, the other approved non-prescription drug, is found in some over-the-counter "appetite" or "weight control" drugs. It supposedly numbs taste, smell or other qualities of food. In my opinion, it does not work.

If you want to try medications for weight control, first join a professional program. Then discuss this possibility with your counselor from that program and consider only prescription medications—if you and your counselor view that option as worthwhile.

Self-Help Programs and Books

You could end a slump by participating in either Take Off Pounds Sensibly (TOPS—**tops.com**) or Weight Watchers (**weightwatchers.com**). These programs cost relatively modest amounts of money. Every major city in the United States and many smaller towns have TOPS chapters (10,000+ nationwide) and Weight Watchers groups that meet frequently. These approaches provide support for change and may help you refocus. Wellspring is currently considering the creation of its own self-help program, Wellspring Journey.

Many self-help books, video tapes, CDs, websites and apps can help you refocus. Materials are available on relaxation, eating, nutrition, depression, visualization and other topics that may re-awaken your commitment to effective weight control. Among the better weight control websites are **calorieking.com**, **weightwatchers.com** and **ediet.com**. *My Fitness Pal* is among the most popular apps for weight controllers.

Professional Help

Hospitals and medical centers sometimes offer programs, such as Optifast (see **www.optifast.com**), that can help more people more of the time than self-help materials or other programs. Look for professionally conducted programs focused on weight loss directed by psychologists with expertise in cognitive-behavioral therapy. Programs that provide help for unlimited periods of time (no less than one year) are especially worthy of consideration. Web searches and calls to local hospitals, colleges and universities (psychology departments), may prove helpful. The following two national organizations have relevant listings of psychologists in virtually every area of the United States: the Association for Behavioral and Cognitive Therapies and the American Psychological Association.

Consumer Reports recently reported on the largest survey ever conducted among people who had obtained professional help for psychological problems other than or in addition to weight loss. More than four thousand readers of that magazine answered twenty-six questions about mental health professionals, family doctors and support groups that they sought for help with psychological distress. Among their most intriguing, and hopeful, findings were:

- People who obtain help from their family doctors tended to feel better after obtaining the help. But people who saw a mental health specialist for more than six months did much better.
- Most people who took medications for psychological problems reported feeling better, but about half of the respondents reported substantial and troublesome side effects (like drowsiness and a feeling of disorientation).
- The longer people stayed in therapy, the more they improved.
- Most people who went to a self-help group (like Alcoholics Anonymous) were very satisfied with the experience and said they got better.
- Almost everyone who sought help experienced some relief, but people who started out feeling the worst reported the most progress.

Mental health professionals define depression as including at least five of the following problems for at least two weeks. At least one of the problems must be either depressed mood or loss of interest in pleasure:

1. Depressed mood, most of the day, nearly every day
2. Markedly less interest or pleasure in all, or almost all, activities most of the day, nearly every day
3. Significant weight loss or weight gain when not dieting, or increase in appetite, nearly every day
4. Insomnia or hypersomnia (excess sleeping), nearly every day
5. Excess physical movement or slowing down in physical movements, nearly every day
6. Fatigue or loss of energy, every day
7. Feelings of worthlessness or excessive or inappropriate guilt, nearly every day
8. Decreased ability to think or concentrate, or indecisiveness, nearly every day
9. Recurrent thoughts of death (not just fear of dying), recurrent suicidal thoughts without a specific plan or suicide attempt or specific plan for committing suicide

Many people experience significant depressions and other forms of psychological distress at some point in their lives. You can imagine how depression can interfere with successful weight control. When feeling depressed, people struggle to stay focused on almost anything in their lives, let alone something as difficult as becoming a successful weight controller. I have heard many people say, "I just didn't care." This statement often accompanies significant lapses or slumps. Unfortunately, once again, your biology has no sympathy. If you feel lousy, for whatever reason, your biology will be more than happy to add excess pounds.

People try many things to get out of depression and other unpleasant psychological states. You can try talking to close friends, taking vacations or changing something significant in your life. When all of your best efforts do not produce positive change, consider taking the next step. You can seek professional help for marital problems or problems with your moods, such as depression. You can ask close friends or relatives for referrals to licensed professionals in your area whom they know or have heard good things about. You can also call your local hospital or university and ask how to get professional assistance.

Most health insurance policies cover substantial amounts of the costs involved with such treatment. Most communities also provide relatively low-cost counseling. You can find these services by calling your place of worship or your local mental health association.

If at all possible, try to find a therapist who is licensed in your state and either a psychologist, social worker or psychiatrist. Psychologists receive five to eight years of training beyond a bachelor's degree. This training focuses on the scientific aspects of helping people change. Social workers receive one to three years of training beyond a bachelor's degree, focused on how to form good relationships with people and to understand resources available in communities that can prove helpful. Psychiatrists receive a medical degree and then several years of training beyond that to help them specialize in how to help people with significant problems in their lives.

Psychiatrists are the only mental health professionals who can prescribe medications for psychological problems in most states. Several states currently allow some psychologists to prescribe medications now, too. Unfortunately, many psychiatrists prescribe medications too quickly. You can find yourself being treated with a powerful set of medications (with sometimes complicated side effects) while other, less chemical methods can produce better outcomes. Therefore, I recommend seeing a licensed psychologist or social worker before seeing a psychiatrist. If medications seem like they would be helpful to you, these other licensed mental health professionals will certainly recommend that you get a consultation from a psychiatrist in order to use such treatments. I believe that if you can find a way of changing without using medications, you will achieve better results and feel better in the long run.

Many weight controllers who become depressed delay getting help. Certainly problems take a while to resolve on your own. You may ask friends or family for help. You may read about the problem and attempt to change yourself. These efforts are worthy of admiration and respect. If and when they do not produce positive outcomes, however, please take action quickly. Your biology acts very rapidly to cause you trouble. A lapse can turn into a slump. To avoid this downward spiral, *action* must become your middle name. Your biology does not allow you to stay in a slump very long without punishing you much more severely than the person who doesn't struggle with weight problems.

Sports psychologists provide very similar advice to elite athletes. When athletes struggle with emotional issues, their performances decline, just as your weight increases. Performance declines can rapidly become major slumps. Major slumps can ruin careers. Athletes and weight controllers must take action quickly to grapple with whatever problems face them. Quick actions on the part of athletes can end slumps. The same applies to you.

RATIONAL EMOTIVE THERAPY (RET) PRINCIPLES

Thus far, this chapter emphasized understanding common stressors and the value of developing active methods of coping to master those challenges. Located in between recognizing challenges and taking action is the way you think about yourself and the world. Negative thoughts can lead to depressed and anxious moods. In this way, they could easily prevent you from taking critical action steps. Let's consider a very powerful way to help you shift your moods by modifying the way you think. More constructive actions can follow when your moods stay more consistently upbeat. You can, indeed, become undisturbable. To develop the thinking skills to allow you to reach such a lofty goal, however, takes some practice. This again resembles most athletic challenges. If you can learn the way to think yourself to an undisturbable stance, then the payoff can take your weight control game to a much higher level.

Shakespeare wrote something about this in *Hamlet*: "There's nothing either good or bad but thinking makes it so."

Introduction to RET

Psychologist Albert Ellis agreed with Shakespeare about this. Our thoughts powerfully influence our moods. In the 1950s, Dr. Ellis realized that the existing methods of helping people improve their moods, primarily psychoanalysis (a Freudian approach), did not work very well. He created a new approach based on analyzing the quality of thinking and how to change it. In order to take the actions described early in this chapter, sometimes you will benefit from viewing yourself or your situation differently. To do this, you will find using Ellis' Rational Emotive Therapy (RET) principles remarkably helpful. RET can help you change your thinking and, as a consequence, change your moods and actions.

RET takes the position that the world includes a series of positive, negative and neutral events. Our thoughts interpret those events. Thoughts essentially create feelings much more so than the actual events. If a weight controller saw the same number on a scale on Tuesday as Monday, then that weight controller might view that event as horrible and become very agitated (sad, frustrated). Another person in the exact same situation might consider that stability a neutral or even positive event. From an RET perspective, therefore:

WORLD -> THOUGHTS -> MOODS

Stinkin' Thinkin'

What kinds of thoughts make you sad or anxious? Think about the last time you felt either of those negative emotions. Can you trace backwards from the emotions to the thoughts? Most people struggle to do that. Albert Ellis, Aaron Beck and other theorists and researchers found that thoughts that decreased people's sense of hopefulness or control caused unhappy moods. They referred to such problematic thoughts as "irrational thoughts." Albert Ellis also called this "stinkin' thinkin.'" Sometimes RET practitioners use the term "automatic thoughts" to describe this kind of stinkin' thinkin'. Take a look at the following examples and see if you can detect how and why thinking them could create problems:

- Everyone should love me.
- Every problem has an ideal solution.
- I have to be highly competent in everything I do.
- Other people should always treat me considerately and fairly.
- I must lose weight every week.
- If I don't lose weight every week, then I'm a failure—and I may as well give up.
- If I don't succeed every week, then my group leader and members will think I am worthless, a failure and uncommitted; so I may as well give up.
- If I don't eat the food my host offers me, she will hate me.
- I should not deprive my family of treats just because I am trying to lose weight.

What common elements did you observe in these irrational thoughts? Can you see the decreased sense of control some of them imply? For example, "I must lose weight…" and "I have to be highly competent…" demand a certain outcome with no wiggle room for alternatives. Some of these statements also engender hopelessness. The two statements that have "I may as well give up" at their conclusion certainly make that point clear.

The language within your thoughts provides cues that you can use to find your tendency to think in problematic terms. Certain words tell the story. Table 11-3 summaries the types of extreme and absolute words that can help identify irrational or *automatic problematic thoughts* (APTs). Extreme words tend to exaggerate ideas and events, sometimes creating a sense of hopelessness. Absolute words, sometimes called "categorical imperatives," demand certain actions or outcomes. They tend to limit our sense of choice and control. Both hopelessness and feeling out of control can cause depressed or anxious feelings.

You can take several steps to examine the effects of these problematic thoughts in your life. First, try to go an entire day without using any of the absolute words listed in Table 11-3, both in what you say to others and also what you say to yourself. You will find it very challenging to do this. Particularly try to avoid using the word "should" when talking to yourself or others.

In order to give yourself a good chance to succeed at this challenge, it would help you to know the likely and best alternatives to use instead of such words. Try substituting an expression of preference or desire instead. For example, decide what you can say to modify the following

Table 11-3
Extreme and Absolute Words

Extreme Words	Absolute Words
All	Have to
Awful	Need
Essential	Must
Every	Ought
Horrible	Should
Terrible	
Totally	

statement to eliminate use of the word "should": "Everyone should love me." Instead of "should," you can express a preference. For example, "I'd prefer it if everyone loved me, but I know that's impossible." Or, "I like it when people seem to like me, but I know that's not going to happen with everyone."

EAT:
Emotion, Automatic Problematic Thoughts and Turn-Around Thoughts

Exercise 11-2 helps you track the use of these APTs and learn how to turn them around with alternative thoughts (turn-around thoughts). Any time you experience a negative emotion for the next week, try entering it into this exercise and re-working your reaction to the situation that caused the APT.

If you do this for several weeks, then you will take a huge step toward becoming more undisturbable. For additional examples, see the APTs below and the turn-around thoughts following each of them in italics:

- Everyone should love me. *I'd like it if everyone loved me, but I know that's impossible. Some people just don't get along and that's okay.*

- Every problem has an ideal solution. *Problems by definition are challenges without immediately obvious or ideal solutions. Problems often have best solutions, but rarely do they have ideal solutions. For example, my car is getting older and starting to cost more and more money to keep running. I could get another car, but that's a huge expense. Or, I could keep sinking money into it to hope it keeps going for a while longer. Neither solution is ideal; both involve risks. If money is very tight, then keeping the car longer might make more sense, perhaps after getting a mechanic I trust to give me his best guess as to the car's longevity.*

- I have to be highly competent in everything I do. *I'd like to be competent in everything but that's very unlikely. It also depends on my standards for competence. Is bowling 150 competent or does it take 200 consistently to reach that standard? It's just fine if I'm competent at the things that matter most to me and merely okay at others.*

- **Other people should always treat me considerately and fairly.** *I'd like that to happen, but people vary tremendously in the way they treat each other. People also vary in the way they are likely to treat me based on how they feel on a particular day, level of stress and other factors.*

- **I must lose weight every week.** *As a weight controller, I'd like that. It's just unrealistic. So many factors determine the number on the scale. The scale is an imperfect measure of effort. I can control the effort I put into my program and my consistency in key areas, at least to some extent. It's harder to control a number on a scale.*

- **If I don't lose weight every week, then I'm a failure—and I may as well give up.** *I could use a much better standard to determine my success/failure than weight loss every week. For example, I can evaluate my consistency in self-monitoring and reaching my step goals. The process matters too, not just the numbers on the scale.*

- **If I don't succeed every week, then my group leader and members will think I am worthless, a failure and uncommitted; so I may as well give up.** *My group leaders and members are there to support me, not to reject me for being imperfect. They're not going to view me as worthless because I struggle at this difficult task. That would be both mean and unreasonable.*

- **If I don't eat the food my host offers me, she will hate me.** *Hosts don't care that much about what everyone eats. If someone were to hate me because of what I ate or didn't eat, then I wouldn't want her for a friend anyway.*

- **I should not deprive my family of treats just because I am trying to lose weight.** *My family wants to support me. The Wellspring Plan allows for plenty of treats, just ones that are very low in fat and on the program. They'll learn to feel satisfied with Wellspring-friendly treats and their health will improve because of this.*

Exercise 11-2
EAT: Changing Your Thinking to Improve Your Moods

Instructions: Use this form to track your negative emotions and identify the automatic problematic thoughts (APTs) associated with them. Highlight the key problematic word/words. Then, in the final column, rewrite those ATPs to make them turn-around thoughts—more constructive, hopeful and positive thoughts. See the two examples in italics and then complete the form with your own entries for this week.

Day/ Time	Emotion	Automatic Problematic Thoughts (APTs)	Turn Around Thoughts
Monday 9am	Frustrated	I **should** have lost weight this week.	I really wanted to lose weight and would have preferred losing weight this week. The scale is an imperfect measure. I know I worked at this because I self-monitored well and met my step goals.
Thursday 7pm	Annoyed	I **hate** when my friends offer me high-fat foods. It's a **horrible** bind that they put me in when they do that.	I'd rather my friends understood my weight control program better than they do; but this isn't a hateful act on their part. The bind I'm in is challenging, not horrible.

Day/Time	Emotion	Automatic Problematic Thoughts (APTs)	Turn Around Thoughts

CONCLUSIONS

This chapter began by considering the concept of strength of self-regulation, essentially arguing that we have limited resources for such challenges as weight control. If we can learn to manage the stressful aspects of our lives more efficiently, then we'll feel more energized to continue progress as weight controller-athletes. The chapter reviewed concepts related to this quest, from stressors to stress management, high-risk situations to slumps and slump busters. Finally, we reviewed RET principles, particularly emphasizing the value of the EAT exercise.

No one manages weight control perfectly. It's just too demanding a taskmaster, requiring the taming of resistant biology in the context of an obesogenic culture. Yet, we can do our best to execute the seven steps of the Wellspring Plan, keeping in sharp focus the 3-1-7 nature of it (3 simple behavioral goals [0 fat g; 12,000 steps; 100 percent self-monitoring]), one overarching mission (healthy obsession) and seven steps to success (from knowing the biology to making the decision to becoming undisturbable). The effort demands a lot, but it gives back even more. The case studies in the first chapter documented this in human terms. I've watched thousands transform themselves in clinic offices and through Wellspring's immersion CBT programs. Weight controllers almost always get help from others along the way, and those others quite often get healthier in the process too. I'm hoping that you and yours will join this healthier and happier collective. The final part of this book provides specifics about food to help you do exactly that.

In 1958, obesity expert Albert Stunkard summarized the research from the previous thirty years of scientific efforts to control obesity by saying, "Most obese persons will not stay in treatment for obesity. Of those who stay in treatment, most will not lose weight, and of those who do lose weight, most will regain it."

The principles in this book suggest much greater optimism about how to manage this very tricky problem. This book is based on science. That science provides you with hope, if you understand that you are a weight controller-athlete and then follow the key principles described here. You can lose weight and keep it off if you are willing to understand the evidence provided by science and stay in the struggle, no matter what—to use the three simple behavioral goals, Wellspring's seven steps, and nurture your healthy obsession. The recent research on people who use these principles provides a clear basis for hope:

- Only 12 percent of people involved in the 1928-1958 research lost twenty pounds or more; in recent studies that percent has quadrupled: approximately 50 percent of those in the best treatment programs now lose twenty pounds or more.

- Results from participants in professional programs that use very restricted calorie intake and professional counseling show that 90 percent of people in such treatments lose twenty pounds or more and that 50 percent lose forty pounds or more, compared with only 1 percent in the research conducted in the first half of the twentieth century.

- In some immersion CBT programs most participants lose twenty pounds or more and many maintain substantial weight losses for many years. For example, in 2012, the average Wellspring camper who participated for at least six weeks lost twenty-seven pounds. Wellspring follow-up studies (six to eighteen months) repeatedly have shown that about one third of participants continue losing weight after going home (quite a few lose fifty pounds or more) and another third maintain those substantial weight losses for at least a year, sometimes for many years.

PART 4
Foodstuffs

CHAPTER 12

Dietary Tips for Following the Wellspring Plan

Now we'll review ideas, developed and tested in Wellspring's programs for the past ten years, focused on how to maintain a very low-fat diet in the most enjoyable and satisfying way. It includes very low-fat substitutes for commonly used high-fat foods, very low-fat cooking tips, quick and easy ideas for meals and snacks and recommendations for how to stock your cupboard. Finally, you will find dozens of the favorite recipes developed by Wellspring's chefs that thousands of campers and their families have enjoyed at Wellspring's programs and at home.

Very Low-Fat Substitutes

Recipe calls for:	Substitute:	Cooking Techniques and Other Tips
MEAT		Broil, boil, bake, grill or poach meat. Make lean choices and remove visible fat before cooking.
beef	buffalo, ostrich, emu	
ground beef	ground turkey, chicken or buffalo	
chicken	skinless chicken breast	
canned tuna	water-packed tuna	
DAIRY		
whole milk dairy products	fat-free dairy products	

Recipe calls for:	Substitute:	Cooking Techniques and Other Tips
regular cheese	fat-free cheese	
ricotta cheese	fat-free ricotta	This works great in lasagna.
heavy cream	2 tablespoons flour + 2 cups fat-free milk	
whipped cream	evaporated skim milk, chilled	
sour cream	fat-free sour cream	
mayonnaise	fat-free mayonnaise	
FATS/OILS		
butter or oil for baking	applesauce, pureed fruits (like prunes) or pureed vegetables	Use 1 cup of the substitution for every cup of butter/oil in the recipe. It is better to use unsweetened applesauce. If sweetened applesauce is used, reduce sugar/sweetener by $1/3$. Pureed prunes work well in recipes with chocolate.
butter or oil for browning	non-stick spray, fat-free broth, wine, herbs and seasonings	Use 3 tablespoons fat-free broth or wine for every 1 tablespoon butter or oil called for in recipe.
VEGETABLES	Cook with herbs, lemon and lime juice and fat-free broth instead of fat	Steam, stir fry
EGGS	1 ½ large egg whites or ¼ cup egg substitute	

Very Low-Fat Cooking Tips

Here are some basic tips to help you make very low-fat choices when cooking.

Meats

- Bake, broil, grill or steam lean meat and poultry.
- When roasting or grilling meat, place on a rack to allow the fat to drain.
- Choose lean meats like fish and chicken.
- Always remove skin from poultry and trim fat from meats before cooking.
- Use marinades to tenderize lean cuts of meat. Make fat-free choices like red wine vinegar, juice, wine, soy sauce and herbs.

Veggies

- Stir fry vegetables in fat-free broth, water, lemon/lime juice or light soy sauce.
- Make grilled kabobs using lean meat and vegetable chunks.
- Add fat-free yogurt or sour cream to potatoes.
- Squeeze lemon/lime or add pepper to steamed veggies.
- Char-grill veggies right on the grill or wrap in foil.

In General

- Use vegetable oil cooking sprays, lemon or lime juice or broth in place of oil whenever possible.
- Skim fat from homemade soups by chilling and removing the fat layer that rises to the surface.
- Flavor enhancing ingredients:
    - Herbs, spices, garlic, vinegar, ginger, mustard, lemon juice, wine, soy sauce, hot sauce and salsa.

QUICK AND EASY BREAKFAST IDEAS

These ideas can help you create healthy breakfasts that you can grab when you don't have time to cook:

- High-fiber cereal with skim milk and fresh or frozen fruit
- Fat-free yogurt with fruit and/or high-fiber cereal
- Whole grain toast with:
    Reduced sugar jam and fat-free cream cheese or fat-free ricotta
    ½ mashed banana and cinnamon
- Lean ham or turkey and fat-free cottage cheese or cheddar
- Plain instant oatmeal or oatmeal with sliced banana and cinnamon
- Fat-free cottage cheese with tomatoes or other fruit
- Scrambled eggs made from fat-free egg beaters, fat-free cheese and veggies (chop veggies the night before)
- 1 low-fat bran muffin (make enough on the weekend for breakfast and snacks during the week)
- 1 or 2 low-fat pancakes or waffles served with fruit (make enough on the weekend for breakfast and snacks during the week)

- Wheat bagel with fat-free cream cheese (<210 calories per whole bagel, not the huge 6 oz. bagels that can have 500 calories or more)

QUICK AND EASY DINNER IDEAS

Here are some dinner ideas you can use after a long day that will help your family stay healthy. It's all in the preparation:
- If you grill meat on the weekend, prepare an extra batch, slice and refrigerate for meals later in the week.
- Bagged salad greens cut down on preparation time.
- Make fat-free chili on the weekends and freeze for snacks and meals throughout the week.

Chicken or beef (very lean, buffalo preferred) dinners:
- Chicken/beef fajitas: fill a wheat pita with chicken and veggies sautéed with your choice of wine, herbs, vinegar, ginger, garlic, lemon or soy sauce. Add fat-free cheese if desired.
- Wrap chicken breast, salsa, corn and beans in tin foil and bake. Serve with brown rice or on a wheat tortilla.
- Warm chicken/beef and use it to top a salad with fat-free dressing and tons of veggies.
- Add chicken to pasta with fat-free marinara sauce (substitute some pasta with fresh green beans for variety).

Very low-fat or veggie chili can be used as:
- A great baked potato topper with fat-free cheese.
- A low-fat tortilla filler with cooked veggies.

Other ideas:
- Try grilled, baked or steamed fish/chicken and veggies with brown rice.
- In the morning: fill a crockpot with chicken breast or buffalo, your choice of vegetables and seasoning (wine, herbs, juice, etc.). Add enough liquid to make a soup.
- Small sweet potatoes take about five minutes in the microwave. Top with fat-free, sugar-free vanilla yogurt and/or cinnamon. Sweet potatoes are also a great veggie with chicken or pork tenderloin dishes.

- For vegetarian dishes, add whole grain toast with fat-free cheese.
- Idaho potatoes with fat-free cheese and broccoli.

HIGH-FIBER SNACKS

Fiber is important to include in snacks because it can help increase feelings of fullness. Here are some ideas to get more fiber out of your snacks:

- Eat whole grain toast with a slice of lean meat and mustard.
- Mix different kinds of dry cereal for flavor and a granola-like snack.
- Try a fat-free dip with raw veggies like broccoli, green peppers, carrots or green beans.
  - Mix dry ranch mix, dry green onion mix or any other dry fat-free seasoned mix with fat-free sour cream for a tasty dip.
- Cut up fresh fruit like apples, berries, oranges, peaches and pears and serve with fat-free yogurt or cottage cheese.
- Air-popped popcorn makes a great snack. Add seasonings (but not butter).
- Try fat-free string cheese and a half of a small apple.
- For a cold treat: eat frozen grapes or berries.

But remember, all of these foods are not limitless and calories count. The following are serving sizes for 100-calorie snacks and some limitless snacks.

100-Calorie Snacks	Serving Size
Dry Cereal	½–¾ cup
Fat-free dip with ½ cup raw veggies	¼ cup
Fat-free cottage cheese or yogurt with ½ small piece of fruit or ½ cup berries	½ cup
Air-popped popcorn	3 cups
Fat-free string cheese + ½ small apple	1 each
Frozen grapes	1½ cup
Frozen berries	1 cup

Limitless Snacks

- Asparagus
- Bean/Alfalfa sprouts
- Broccoli
- Cabbage
- Celery
- Cucumbers
- Herbs
- Jicama
- Lemon
- Lettuce
- Mushrooms
- Onions
- Peppers
- Pickles
- Radishes
- Tomatoes

Stocking Your Cupboard: Recommended Staples

CONDIMENTS

- Fat-Free Mayonnaise
- Peanut Butter Substitute
- Fat-Free Parmesan Cheese
- Spicy Mustard
- Balsamic Vinaigrette
- Light Soy Sauce
- Barbeque Sauce
- Teriyaki Sauce
- Fat-Free Salad Dressings
- Fat-Free Cooking Sauces
- Dill Pickles
- Sucralose-based artificial sweetener
- Sucralose Baking Sugar
- Sucralose Brown Sugar
- Capers
- Roasted Red Peppers
- Garlic Salt
- Seasoning Salt
- Old Bay Seasoning
- Ground Cumin
- Curry Powder
- Dried Thyme
- Dried Rosemary
- Allspice
- Cinnamon
- Non-Fat No-Calorie Cooking Spray

DAIRY

- Fat-Free Sour Cream
- Fat-Free Milk
- Fat-Free, Sugar-Free Vanilla Yogurt
- Fat-Free Plain Yogurt
- Fat-Free Cottage Cheese
- Fat-Free Cream Cheese
- Fat-Free Cheddar Cheese
- Fat-Free American Cheese
- Fat-Free Ricotta Cheese

Fat-Free Feta Cheese
Egg Substitute
Egg White Substitute
Fat-Free Buttermilk

Fat-Free, Sugar-Free Ice Cream
Butter-Spray (Non-Fat)
Fat-Free, Sugar-Free Whipped Topping

DRY GOODS

Whole Wheat Pasta—angel hair, manicotti shells, macaroni
Whole Wheat Flour
Panko Bread Crumbs
Whole Wheat Bread Crumbs
Instant Oatmeal
Fat-Free Pretzels
Raisins
Beef Jerky
Fat-Free Brownie Mix
Caramel Corn Rice Cakes
Fat-Free Potato Chips
Baked Tortilla Chips
Salsa

Canned Beans
Low-Fat Tortillas
Sugar-Free Pudding Mix
Angel Food Cake
Brown Rice
Canned Vegetables
Canned Fruit in juice
Fat-Free Drink Mix
Canned Tuna in water
Canned Tomatoes (Diced, sauce, paste)
Tomato Juice
Chicken and Vegetable Broths
Fat-Free Canned Soups
Low-Fat, High-fiber Cereals

MEATS

Lean Deli Meats (Turkey, Ham, Chicken)
Boneless, Skinless Chicken Breast
Lean Buffalo Meat 97 percent meat to 3 percent fat
Lean Turkey Meat 97 percent meat to 3 percent fat

Roasted Turkey Breast (Skinless)
Pork Tenderloin
Lean Fish—tilapia, orange roughy
Shrimp

FAVORITE WELLSPRING RECIPES

BREAKFAST

CREPES

Ingredients
- 4 ounces skim milk
- 4 ounces water
- 3 ounces flour
- 2 ounces egg substitute
- 1.5 tsp. vegetable oil

Method
1. Combine all ingredients into a bowl and mix until smooth.
2. Allow to rest for twenty minutes.
3. To make each crepe: Ladle two tablespoons of the batter into a crepe pan, cook on the first side until the edges look dry.
4. Turn the crepe once and cook briefly on the second side.

Yield: Twelve crepes, six servings of two each

Nutritional Information
- Calories   75
- Protein   3 grams
- Fat   1.3 grams
- Carbs   12 grams

STRAWBERRY BLINTZES

Ingredients
- 12 crepes
- 12 ounces fat-free cream cheese
- 2 ounces skim milk
- ½ tsp. almond extract
- 24 ounces strawberries, fresh

Method
1. Prepare Crepes.

2. Soften fat-free cream cheese in a microwave oven (30 seconds on high).
3. Combine fat-free cream cheese, skim milk, and almond extract. Mix well.
4. Place one ounce of cream cheese mixture in each crepe.
5. Roll crepes and place on a 2" baking dish.
6. Top with 2 ounces of fresh strawberries.
7. Place crepes in a 250 degree oven and warm for 15 minutes.

Yield: 12 crepes, 6 servings, 2 crepes per serving

Nutritional Information
Calories   100
Fat   .5 grams
Protein   4.3 grams
Carbs   5 grams

POTATO PANCAKES

Ingredients
- 2.5 pounds potatoes
- 4 ounces onions (chopped)
- 2.5 ounces egg substitute
- 1.5 ounces flour
- ½ tsp. salt
- ¼ tsp. baking powder
- 1 ounce skim milk

Method
1. Peel and shred potatoes.
2. Chop onions.
3. In a mixing bowl combine potatoes, onion, egg substitute, flour, salt, baking powder and non-fat milk.
4. Heat griddle or frying pan to 350 degrees.
5. Pour three ounces of mixture onto griddle and turn after 3-4 minutes.
6. Remove from griddle when pancakes are golden brown.

Yield: 16 pancakes, 8 servings, two pancakes per serving

Nutritional Information
Calories   114
Protein   4.5 grams
Fat   0 grams
Carbs   23 grams

FRENCH TOAST

Ingredients
- 4 pieces of multigrain or similar whole grain bread
- 4 Tbs. egg whites
- 2 tsp. skim milk
- Dash of vanilla
- Dash of nutmeg

Method
1. Mix wet ingredients in a shallow bowl.
2. Lightly spray skillet and heat on stovetop at medium heat.
3. When skillet is ready, lay bread slices in bowl one at a time so that each side is coated with mixture and place on skillet.
4. Turn bread over after a few minutes (as soon as toast is browned) and heat second side until it is browned.
5. Serve with maple syrup and fat-free vanilla yogurt.

Yield: 2—2 slice servings

Nutritional Information
Calories   164
Protein   4 grams
Fat   2 grams
Carbs   32.5 grams

SPOTTED DOG

Ingredients
- 1 cup brown rice
- ¼ cup raisins
- ¼ tsp. cinnamon
- 1 Tbs. brown sugar
- 2 Tbs. skim milk
- 2 cups water

Method
1. Mix rice, raisins, cinnamon and sugar in a side bowl.
2. Bring 2 cups of water to a boil, then add ingredients to water.
3. Return to boil and then simmer for 20 minutes until most of the water is evaporated.
4. Add milk (more if a creamier mixture is desired).

Yield: 4—1 cup servings

Nutritional Information
Calories   225 calories
Protein   9 grams
Fat   1.5 grams
Carbs   43.9 grams

FRITTATA

Ingredients
- 2 cups onion
- 3 cups broccoli
- 1 sliced mushroom
- Dash of thyme
- ¾ tsp. black pepper
- 3 cups egg whites
- 1 cup fat-free Mozzarella cheese

Method
1. Lightly spray fat-free cooking spray in a skillet and heat on medium.
2. Sauté onions until clear.

3. Add broccoli and continue to sauté for 4-5 minutes; add mushrooms and cook until soft.
4. Sprinkle with thyme and black pepper.
5. Reduce heat to medium-low and pour egg over vegetables.
6. Turn heat to low and continue to heat.
7. As eggs solidify sprinkle cheese on top.
8. Heat on stovetop until edges begin to firm.
9. Place in oven at 350 degrees until center is firm.

Yield: 8–1 cup servings

Nutritional Information
Calories   94
Protein   18 grams
Fat   0 grams
Carbs   5.5 grams

LUNCH

PITA POCKET PIZZA

Ingredients
6-inch fat-free pita pockets
2 ounces fat-free pizza sauce
6 ounces fat-free jack cheese
6 ounces fat-free cheddar cheese

Method
1. Place pita pocket on a clean surface.
2. Spread two ounces of pizza sauce on each pocket.
3. Top with one ounce of fat-free jack cheese and fat-free cheddar cheese.
4. Sprinkle cheese with water.
5. Place in 350 degree oven for 10-15 minutes.

Yield: 6 Servings

Nutritional Information
Calories   260
Protein   25 grams
Fat   0 grams
Carbs   40 grams

PIZZA MEXICANA

Ingredients
4 fat-free flour soft taco tortillas
8 ounces fat-free refried beans
3 each fresh tomatoes
8 ounces fat-free jack cheese

Method
1. Place soft tacos on a cookie sheet.
2. Spread 2 ounces of the refried beans on each taco.
3. Dice tomatoes and place on top of the refried beans.
4. Top with 2 ounces of fat-free jack cheese.
5. Sprinkle cheese with a small amount of water.
6. Bake in a 350 degree oven until cheese "melts."

Yield: 4 servings (1 taco each)

Nutritional Information
Calories   232
Fat   .18 grams
Protein   23.5 grams
Carbs   35 grams

GRILLED MANDARIN CHICKEN PITA SANDWICH

Ingredients
- 1 pound of boneless, skinless chicken breast
- 4 whole wheat pitas
- 2 cups mandarin oranges (canned in water)
- 2 cups chopped romaine lettuce
- 2 Tbs. chopped chives
- 2 Tbs. low-calorie, no oil Italian dressing
- 1 tsp. soy sauce

Method
1. Preheat grill to 350 degrees.
2. Grill chicken breasts until done, then put them in the refrigerator to cool.
3. Combine Italian dressing, soy sauce and chopped chives then set aside.
4. Cut grilled chicken breast in cubes and add to dressing. Let marinate for 30 minutes.
5. After marinated, add full contents of dressing and chicken to chopped romaine and mandarin oranges in a bowl then toss until evenly coated.
6. Cut pita into halves and open them into pockets.
7. Add lettuce mixture to pockets and serve.

Yield: 4 servings (1 stuffed pita each)

Nutritional Information
Calories   310.25
Protein   29.45 grams
Fat   2.9 grams
Carbs   41.6 grams

VEGETARIAN LASAGNA

Ingredients
- 1-10 oz. package of lasagna noodles
- 32 oz. fat-free ricotta cheese (32 oz. fat-free cottage cheese may be substituted, but must be drained)
- ⅓ cup of egg substitute or egg whites
- 3 green onions, diced
- 2 cups of pre-made, pasta sauce
- 1 medium yellow/red/green pepper, chopped
- 1-10 oz. bag frozen spinach, thawed
- 2 cups fat-free Mozzarella cheese
- ½ cup fat-free Parmesan cheese

Method
1. Pre-heat oven to 350 F.
2. Cook lasagna noodles according to the instructions printed on packaging until noodles are firm.
3. Mix together ricotta cheese, egg substitute and diced onions in a medium bowl.
4. Layer cooked noodles, Ricotta mixture and sauce, adding vegetables and ½ of the Mozzarella in periodically, into a 12 x 14 inch baking pan.
5. Top layers with remaining Mozzarella and Parmesan cheese.
6. Cover pan with tin foil and bake lasagna for 1 hour (remove foil for the last 15 minutes so that top layer is slightly browned).

Yield: 12—6 ounces (¾ cup) servings

Nutritional Ingredients:

Calories	156
Protein	12 grams
Fat	0.6 grams
Carbs	25.6 grams

DINNER

BUFFALO STEW

Ingredients
- 2 lbs. bison stew meat
- 2 lbs. red potatoes
- 2 stalks celery
- ½ gallon water
- 1 lb. carrots
- 8 ounces onions
- 1.5 tsp. Worcestershire sauce
- 2 cloves garlic
- 1.5 tsp. paprika

Method
1. Brown the buffalo meat on high heat (about 3 minutes).
2. Combine all ingredients except vegetables.

3. Cover and cook on low heat for 3 hours.
4. Add vegetables and cook for an additional 30 minutes.
5. Adjust flavor and color by adding beef base.
6. For a thicker sauce add cornstarch until attaining desired texture.

Yield: 6—12 oz. servings

Nutritional Information
Calories 204
Protein 9 grams
Fat 1.87 grams
Carbs 37.5 grams

BUFFALO MEATLOAF

Ingredients
1.5 lbs. ground bison
2 slices bread, crumbled
½ cup skim milk
2.5 ounces egg substitute
1 ounce onion (chopped)
1.5 tsp. table salt
1.5 tsp. pepper

Method
1. Combine all ingredients in a mixing bowl.
2. At low speed, mix ingredients until blended.
3. Pour ingredients into a small loaf pan.
4. Bake at 325 degrees for 1.5 hours.

Yield: 6—6 oz. servings

Nutritional Information
Calories 160
Protein 26 grams
Fat 2.12 grams
Carbs 9.25 grams

GINGER PINEAPPLE CHICKEN STIR FRY WITH SNOW PEAS

Ingredients
1 pound boneless, skinless chicken breast
1 red bell pepper
1 cup fresh pineapple chunks
2 cups fresh snow peas
¾ cup sliced shiitake mushrooms
1 red onion rough chopped
1 Tbs. chopped garlic
1 Tbs. minced fresh ginger
½ cup soy sauce
1 Tbs. sesame seeds

Method
1. Spray non-stick frying pan with a non-fat cooking spray. Add

to pan sesame seeds, chopped garlic and chicken strips. Sauté for 2 minutes.
2. Add red pepper, onion, ginger and mushrooms. Continue to sauté for 1 minute.
3. Add soy sauce, pineapple, red pepper flakes and snow peas. Cover and let cook for 1 minute.
4. Uncover and stir until chicken and vegetables are covered

with sauce and chicken is fully cooked.

Yield: 4—8 oz. servings

Nutritional Information
Calories   243
Protein   29.93 grams
Fat   3.68 grams
Carbs   22.5 grams

SOUR CREAM CHICKEN

Ingredients
1.25 lbs. boneless, skinless chicken breast
1 cup onions, chopped
5 Tbs. paprika
½ tsp. salt
2 cups fat-free chicken broth
2 cups fat-free sour cream
2 tsp. flour

Method
1. Lightly spray pan (oven safe dish) with cooking spray and place chicken breasts in pan.
2. Bake in a 350 degree oven for 20 minutes.
3. Sauté onions in a skillet (use cooking spray) until translucent, not brown.
4. Add chicken broth, paprika and salt—reduce stove to low heat.
5. Stir flour into the sour cream, mix well.
6. Slowly add sour cream mixture to the broth, mix well.
7. Add reserved chicken breasts and simmer until chicken is heated through and the sauce has thickened.

Yield: 5—4 oz. servings

Nutritional Information
Calories   201
Protein   31 grams
Fat   1.66 grams
Carbs   15.5 grams

CHICKEN NUGGETS

Ingredients
- 12 ounces boneless, skinless chicken breast
- 1 cup corn flakes
- 1 tsp. paprika
- ½ tsp. Italian herb seasoning
- 1 tsp. garlic powder
- ¼ tsp. onion powder
- ½ tsp. salt

Method
1. Cut chicken breasts into bite-sized pieces.
2. Place cornflakes in plastic bag and crush by using a rolling pin.
3. Add remaining ingredients to crushed cornflakes. Close bag and shake until blended.
4. Add a few chicken pieces at a time to crumb mixture. Shake to coat evenly.
5. Lightly spray a cooking sheet.
6. Heat oven to 400 degrees.
7. Place chicken pieces on cooking sheet so they are not touching.
8. Bake until golden brown, about 12-14 minutes.

Yield: 4—3.25 oz. servings

Nutritional Information
- Calories 168
- Protein   27 grams
- Fat   3.13 grams
- Carbs   7.75 grams

TERIYAKI CHICKEN KABOBS

Ingredients
- ½ cup Teriyaki marinade
- 1 lb. boneless, skinless chicken
- 1 green bell pepper
- 1 red bell pepper
- 8 mushrooms
- 1 red onion
- 8 cherry tomatoes
- 4—8-inch wooden skewers

Method
1. Soak 8 inch skewers in water.
2. Pour marinade into large bowl.
3. Cut chicken breasts into one ounce portions.
4. Cut bell peppers and onions into one inch pieces.
5. Place chicken and vegetables in the marinade. Marinate for 45 minutes.
6. Build kabobs by stringing chicken and vegetables onto the skewer.
7. Each skewer should contain 4 pieces of chicken.
8. Heat oven to 350 degrees.
9. Place kabobs on a cooking sheet, spray with fat-free cooking spray.
10. Bake for 20 minutes or until chicken is done.

Yield: 4 kabobs, 1 each

Nutritional Information
  Calories   236
  Protein   33 grams
  Fat   4.3 grams
  Carbs   16.3 grams

SALADS

TUNA SALAD

Ingredients
  8 ounces tuna, canned in water, drained
  2.5 ounces fat-free mayonnaise
  1 tsp. sweet pickle relish

Method
  1. Combine all ingredients in a mixing bowl.
  2. Chill for 45 minutes.

Yield: 4—2 ounce servings

Nutritional Information
  Calories   58
  Protein   10 grams
  Fat   .37 grams
  Carbs: 2 grams

EGG SALAD

Ingredients
  8 ounces egg substitute
  2 ounces fat-free mayonnaise
  ⅛ tsp. white pepper
  ½ tsp. red wine vinegar

Method
  1. Scramble egg substitute according to package directions.
  2. Cool eggs for 30 minutes.
  3. Combine egg substitute, mayonnaise, white pepper and red wine vinegar.

Yield: 5—2 ounce servings

Nutritional Information
  Calories   30
  Protein   4 grams
  Fat   .06 grams
  Carbs: 2.75 grams

CHINESE CHICKEN SALAD

Ingredients
- 12 ounces boneless, skinless chicken breast
- 10 ounces iceberg lettuce
- 4 ounces cilantro
- 8 green onions
- 1.5 ounces cellophane rice noodles
- 2 Tbs. fat-free Chinese chicken salad dressing

Method
1. Roast or boil chicken breasts until done. Allow to cool.
2. Shred iceberg lettuce, trim cilantro, slice green onions.
3. Toss iceberg, cilantro and green onions.
4. Cut chicken breasts in strips.
5. On a plate place 3 ounces of lettuce mix.
6. Top with 3 ounces of chicken breast.
7. Garnish with cellophane noodles.
8. Drizzle 2 Tbs. of fat-free salad dressing over chicken.

Yield: 4 servings

Nutritional Information
- Calories   239
- Protein   28 grams
- Fat   1.7 grams
- Carbs: 12 grams

SHRIMP LOUIE

Ingredients
- 12 ounces cooked shrimp
- 8 ounces Iceberg lettuce (chopped)
- 8 cherry tomatoes
- 2 ounces asparagus (canned and drained)
- 4 stalks celery
- 8 Tbs. fat-free Thousand Island dressing

Method
1. Place cooked shrimp in a colander and rinse thoroughly.
2. On a dinner sized plate spread 2 ounces of chopped lettuce.
3. Place three ounces of shrimp on top of lettuce.
4. Garnish with cherry tomatoes, asparagus and celery.
5. Drizzle 1 ounce of fat-free Thousand Island dressing on each plate.

Yield: 4—4 oz. servings

Nutritional Information
- Calories   191
- Protein   19 grams
- Fat   1.8 grams
- Carbs   24.5 grams

GRILLED ASPARAGUS AND SWEET PEPPER SALAD

Ingredients
- 1 pound fresh asparagus spears
- 1 medium orange bell pepper
- 1 small or medium red onion
- 1 lemon
- 1 lime
- 1 orange
- ¼ cup vinegar
- 2 Tbs. Dijon mustard

Method
1. Preheat grill to 375 degrees.
2. Prepare vegetables for grilling by trimming off rough ends of asparagus, cutting the pepper in half and removing the seeds and slicing the onion.
3. Grill asparagus for only 2 or 3 minutes (you still want it crunchy). Continue grilling the onion and the pepper until they are flavored but still crunchy. Place in refrigerator to cool down.
4. Zest the lemon, lime and orange and set aside.
5. Squeeze juice from the lemon, lime and orange and set aside.
6. Combine vinegar, Dijon mustard, salt, pepper, citrus juices.
7. Chop the onion and pepper then cut the asparagus into thirds.
8. Combine Dijon vinaigrette, citrus zest and vegetables, then toss until evenly coated.

Yield: 4—6 oz. servings

Nutritional Information
Calories   64.25
Protein   3.18 grams
Fat   .78 grams
Carbs   11.13 grams

SOUPS

SPLIT PEA SOUP

Ingredients
- ½ gallon water
- 8 ounces dry split peas
- 2 stalks celery
- 3 ounces diced onion (about ½ an onion)
- 4 ounces diced carrots
- 2 cloves garlic
- Salt to taste
- Pepper to taste

Method
1. Measure ½ water into a large pot.
2. Add peas, celery, onion, carrots and garlic.
3. Bring entire mixture to a boil; simmer for one hour.
4. Add salt and pepper to taste.

Yield: 8—8 ounce servings

Nutritional Information
Calories   61.75
Protein   5.6 grams
Fat   .01 grams
Carbs   9.8 grams

VEGETARIAN CHILI

Ingredients
1 medium onion, minced
2 cloves garlic, minced
2 ribs celery, finely minced
1 bell pepper, chopped
1 tsp. cumin
1 Tbs. chili powder
1-2 bay leaves
½ tsp. oregano
½ tsp. dried basil
¼ tsp. cinnamon
2—15 oz. cans crushed tomatoes
1 zucchini, roughly chopped
¾ cup mushrooms, washed and chopped
15 oz. can black beans

Method
1. Spray the bottom of a large pan with cooking spray and heat onions, garlic, celery and bell peppers.
2. Cook on medium-high heat until vegetables are softened.
3. Add cumin, chili powder, bay leaves, oregano and basil, and cook for 1-2 minutes longer.
4. Add tomatoes, mushrooms, zucchini and cinnamon.
5. Heat to boiling, then reduce heat to simmer and cook for 1 hour, covered.
6. Stir in beans and cook, uncovered, to desired thickness.
7. Season with salt and pepper to taste.

Yield: 7—1 cup servings

Nutritional Information
Calories   75
Protein   3.3 grams
Fat   0.2 grams
Carbs   14.9 grams

SIDES AND SAUCES

ALL CURRIED UP DIP/SPREAD

Ingredients
2 cups fat-free ricotta cheese
1 cup sweet onion, minced
1 Tbs. curry powder
salt and pepper

Method
1. Spray skillet with non-fat cooking spray and heat over medium heat.

2. Add onions and cook until they become translucent, about 3 minutes.
3. Add the curry powder and cook one minute more. Let cool.
4. Stir curry mixture into the fat-free ricotta cheese. Chill for at least one hour. (This can be made in advance and stored in the refrigerator for up to 3 days.)

Yield: 8—¼ cup servings

Nutritional Information
Calories   63
Protein   8 g
Fat   0 g
Carbs   8 g

APPLE OAT BREAD

Ingredients
1 cup white flour
1 cup wheat flour
1 tsp. baking powder
¾ tsp. salt
1 tsp. baking soda
2 Tbs. brown sugar
2 cups oats
6 Tbs. maple syrup
1⅔ cup fat-free yogurt
1¼ cup of hydrated apple

Method
1. Preheat oven to 350 degrees.
2. Mix dry and wet ingredients separately.
3. Combine until dry mix is completely moistened. It will be a thick, sticky dough.
4. With minimal handling, scoop into bread pan and bake for 30 minutes.

Yield: 6—2 slice servings

Nutritional Information
Calories   288
Protein   5.3 grams
Fat   1.4 grams
Carbs   63.2 grams

MANGO MARINADE/SAUCE

Ingredients
2 cups diced mango (fresh or frozen)
5 tsp. fresh ginger
5 Tbs. brown sugar
10 Tbs. cider vinegar
1 tsp. hot sauce
3 tsp. fresh garlic

Method
1. Puree all ingredients in a food processor.

2. Pour over fish, chicken or sliced tofu and bake.

Yield: 8—¼ cup servings

Nutritional Information
Calories   64
Protein   .4 grams
Fat   0 grams
Carbs   15.6 grams

BABA GANOUJ

Ingredients
2 medium eggplants
2-3 lemons worth of juice
¾ cup Tahini
6 Tbsp. minced garlic
½ cup chopped parsley
2 tsp. salt
½ cup chopped scallions (optional)
Black pepper to taste
1 cup fat-free, plain yogurt

Method
1. Preheat oven to 400 degrees.
2. Cut off the stems of both eggplants and prick each eggplant several times with a fork.
3. Place the eggplants directly onto the oven rack and let eggplants cook for approximately 45 minutes, until the skin is shriveled and the eggplant is soft.
4. Remove eggplants from the oven and set them aside until they are cool enough to handle. In the meantime, cut lemons into quarters, measure out tahini and prepare spices.
5. Then, cut along the length of your eggplants and scoop their cooked insides out.
6. Discard skins and put eggplant into a food processor or blender with remaining ingredients.
7. Blend until smooth and creamy.

Yield: 24—2 oz./2 Tbs. servings

Nutrition Information
Calories   35
Protein   1.2 grams
Fat   1.8 grams
Carbs   3.5 grams

HUMMUS

Ingredients
16 oz. can of chickpeas (garbanzo beans)
4 cloves of minced garlic (more if a stronger taste is desired)
2 Tbs. Tahini paste
2 Tbs. lemon juice

⅓ tsp. cumin
⅓ tsp. black pepper
Dash of red pepper
⅔ tsp. of salt (or to taste)

Method
1. Combine all of the ingredients in a food processor or blender and mix until smooth. It may be necessary to add moisture to the mixture; warm water, fat-free milk or fat-free yogurt are acceptable options.
2. Additional ingredients, such as roasted red peppers, sun-dried tomatoes or herbs may be added for a different twist. This recipe can also be prepared with black beans. Nutrition information will be different.

Yield: 8—2 oz./2 Tbs. servings

Nutritional Information:
Calories   47
Protein   4 grams
Fat   1.7 grams
Carbs   3.95 grams

BAKED CAJUN FRENCH FRIES

Ingredients
2 large white potatoes, cut lengthwise into ½ inch sticks
1 Tbs. egg whites or egg substitute
1 tsp. curry powder
1 tsp. garlic salt

Method
1. Preheat oven to 400 degrees.
2. Spray a large cookie sheet covered with heavy duty aluminum foil with non-fat spray.
3. Cut potatoes into fry-like strips.
4. Place potatoes onto the cookie sheet.
5. Brush potatoes lightly with egg whites.
6. Sprinkle on garlic salt and curry powder, making sure to cover every French fry at least lightly.
7. Arrange potato sticks on a baking sheet in single layer. Bake 30 minutes. Turn over all fries at this point. Cook for another 10 minutes, until the fries become golden brown.

Yield: 3 servings—6 oz. per person

Nutritional Information:
Calories   140
Fat   0 g
Protein   4 g
Carbs   25g

FAT-FREE GARLIC BREAD

Ingredients
- 10 oz. French bread (approximately 2" in width, 1" height)
- 30-40 squirts of fat-free butter spray
- 2 tsp. garlic salt

Method
1. Preheat oven to 350 degrees.
2. Slice the bread lengthwise.
3. Spray liberally with the fat-free butter spray
4. Sprinkle the garlic salt to coat one side lightly.
5. Cook at 400 degrees for 15 minutes, until underside is crispy.

Yield: 5 servings (2 oz. each)

Nutritional Information
Calories	130
Protein	4 grams
Fat	0 grams
Carbs	27 grams

Sweet Potatoes

The state that grows more sweet potatoes than any other in the United States is North Carolina. The North Carolina Sweet Potato Commission provided advice that appears in this section about choosing, using and cooking this wonderful food.

How to Choose

Select firm, well-rounded sweet potatoes with clean, smooth skin. Watch out for soft spots, obvious bruises and signs of decay.

How to Use

Do not refrigerate sweet potatoes unless they are cooked. Cold temperatures can cause them to become bitter. Instead, it works best to store sweet potatoes in a cool (55 degrees F is ideal) and dry place. I use newly purchased sweet potatoes within a week or two if possible.

The North Carolina Sweet Potato Commission recommends using only a stainless steel knife to cut sweet potatoes. They also advise to place them in cold water while preparing them to prevent darkening.

Basic Cooking Advice

To Bake: Prick the skin repeatedly with a fork and bake at 400 degrees for 40-50 minutes (until soft to the touch).

- To microwave: Puncture the skin several times and microwave on high power for 6-8 minutes for an 8-ounce sweet potato.
- To boil: In boiling water, place whole sweet potatoes and cook for about 40 minutes.
- To steam: Bring 1.5" of water to a boil in a steamer. Place whole, unpeeled sweet potatoes in a steam basket and cook until tender (40-50 minutes for an 8-ounce sweet potato). When peeled and cut into 1" cubes as an alternative, they will cook in 30 minutes.
- Uncooked: Peel and cut into sticks and dip into your favorite dip.

Typical Toppings

Many great toppings can enhance the flavor and variety of sweet potatoes. Consider trying these suggestions:

- Salsa, particularly fruit salsas
- Cinnamon-flavored applesauce
- Vanilla-flavored fat-free yogurt with cinnamon
- Fat-free imitation butter spread and cinnamon sugar (cinnamon + sweetener)
- Sweet and sour sauce
- Mandarin oranges with crushed pineapple
- Honey mustard combinations (including honey + Dijon mustard)
- Barbecue sauce
- Veggie chili

Nutritional Information
1—5" x 2" sweet potato, baked in skin
Calories   118
Protein   1 grams
Fat   .1 gram
Carbs   27.7 grams

APPLE BAKED SWEET POTATOES

Ingredients
- 6 medium sweet potatoes
- 3 apples
- ⅓ cup brown sugar
- 1 Tbs. flour
- 1 tsp. salt
- 2 Tbs. orange juice

Method
1. Cook sweet potatoes until soft, peel, cut lengthwise and slice.
2. Peel, slice apples.
3. Combine remaining ingredients.
4. Layer ingredients in casserole—first layer potatoes then apples; add the orange juice.
5. Bake at 350 degrees for 1 hour.

Yield: 6—1 potato + ½ apple servings

Nutritional Information
Calories 219
Protein 2.3 grams
Fat 0 grams
Carbs 52.5 grams

CURRIED SWEET POTATO SALAD WITH FRUIT MEDLEY

Ingredients
- 2 pounds sweet potatoes, peeled, diced
- 1 cup fat-free yogurt
- 1 Tbs. curry powder
- 1 piece (1 inch) fresh ginger root, minced
- 1 tsp. brown sugar
- ¼ cup golden raisins
- ⅛ cup dried cherries
- ⅛ cup black raisins
- 4 green onions, chopped
- Salt, freshly ground pepper

Method
1. Place potatoes in large pot; fill with cold water to cover; heat to a boil; simmer potatoes until tender, about 7 minutes; drain, set aside.
2. Combine yogurt, curry powder, ginger root and brown sugar in medium bowl; add potatoes, fruit, onions and salt and pepper to taste; toss to coat.

Yield: 6—8 oz. servings

Nutritional Information
Calories 150
Protein 5 grams
Fat 0 grams
Carbs 32.5 grams

ORANGE LIME SWEET POTATOES

Ingredients
- 1 cup onion
- 1 tsp. garlic
- 1 lb. sweet potato 1" pieces
- 1 cup orange juice
- ¼ cup lime juice
- Salt, pepper

Method
1. Sauté onion and garlic using a non-fat cooking spray.
2. Add sweet potato and juices to skillet.
3. Heat to boiling.
4. Reduce heat, simmer until sauce thickens.
5. Add salt, pepper to taste.

Yield: 6—4 oz. servings

Nutritional Information
- Calories 67
- Protein 1 gram
- Fat 0 grams
- Carbs 15.75 grams

SIAM SWEET POTATOES

Ingredients
- 1½ lbs. sweet potatoes, peeled and cut into ½-inch pieces
- Non-fat cooking spray
- 1 onion, chopped
- 2 cloves garlic, minced
- 1½ tsp. grated fresh gingerroot
- ½ tsp. Thai curry paste
- 1 can (12 oz.) evaporated skim milk
- ¼ tsp. coconut extract
- ½ cup water
- ½ tsp. (or less) salt
- 1 cup frozen green peas, thawed
- 1 Tbs. grated lemon peel
- 4 cups hot cooked white rice
- ¼ cup chopped fresh cilantro
- 2 Tbs. soy-based low-fat substitute for peanut butter

Method
1. In a large saucepan, cover the sweet potatoes with water and heat until boiling. Cook 10 minutes; drain and set aside.
2. Spray the bottom of a large skillet with non-fat cooking spray; add the onion and sauté until tender.
3. Add the garlic, ginger, curry powder and pepper flakes; cook, stirring occasionally, 3 minutes.
4. Add the cooked sweet potatoes, evaporated milk, coconut extract, water and salt; heat to boiling.
5. Reduce the heat, cover and simmer for 20 minutes or until the potatoes are tender.

6. Remove from the heat and stir in the peas and lemon peel.
7. Place the hot cooked rice in a serving dish and top with the potato mixture; add peanut butter substitute; sprinkle with cilantro and serve.

Yield: 6—8 oz. servings

Nutritional Information
Calories   289
Protein   9.67 grams
Fat   0 grams
Carbs   62.6 grams

SWEET POTATO CAKES

Ingredients
- 2 carrots—shredded
- 1 medium sweet potato—shredded
- ½ cup onions—chopped
- 2 cloves garlic—minced
- ⅓ cup black bean dry dip mix
- ½ cup bread crumbs
- ⅛ tsp. fennel—ground
- ½ tsp. cumin
- ½ tsp. coriander
- ¼ tsp. MSG (monosodium glutamate) flavor enhancer
- ¼ cup egg substitute
- ⅛ tsp. cayenne
- ½ to ⅓ cup rolled oats
- ¼ tsp. sesame seeds
- ½ cup frozen peas
- 1 heaping Tbs. shredded fat-free Mozzarella
- 1 Tbs. dried parsley

Method
1. Mix all ingredients together vigorously. Form into small cakes about 3 to 3½" in diameter.
2. Spray a non-stick frying pan with non-fat spray cooking oil.
3. Cook cakes on medium heat for about 10–15 minutes, turning every few minutes; they should be lightly browned and cooked through.
4. Serve with a dollop of fat-free sour cream and garnish with a bit of parsley.

Yield: 4—6 oz. servings

Nutritional Information
Calories   90
Protein   5 grams
Fat   0 grams
Carbs   17.5 grams

SWEET POTATO CARROT SALAD

Ingredients
- 2 large carrots
- 1 medium sweet potato
- 1 cup raisins
- 1 cup chopped fresh pineapple
- 2 tsp. grated fresh ginger

2 tsp. fat-free mayonnaise
1 tsp. fresh lemon juice
Pinch of salt

Method
1. Shred carrots and sweet potato, set aside.
2. Purée the lemon juice with the mayonnaise and a few chunks of the pineapple and salt.
3. Add the raisins, ginger and remaining pineapple to the shredded carrots and sweet potato.
4. Pour the puréed mixture over this, toss and let marinate for ½ hour.
5. Chill.

Yield: 4—6 oz. servings

Nutritional Information
Calories   186
Protein   2.2 grams
Fat   0 grams
Carbs   44.3 grams

SWEET POTATO PANCAKES

Ingredients
4 cups (packed) coarsely grated sweet potatoes (approx. 1 large or 2 medium)
½ cup grated onion
3-4 Tbs. lemon juice
1 tsp. salt
Black pepper, to taste
6 whipped egg whites
⅓ cup flour
Optional: ¼ cup minced parsley

Method
1. Combine all ingredients and mix well.
2. Spray a non-stick frying pan with non-fat cooking spray and heat.
3. Use a non-slotted spoon to form thin pancakes, patting the batter down; brown on both sides; serve hot with toppings (fat-free sour cream or yogurt; applesauce).

Yield: 4—1 cup (4 pancakes) servings

Nutritional Information
Calories   135
Protein   3 grams
Fat   0 grams
Carbs   30.75 grams

SWEET POTATO PIE

Ingredients
- ¾ cup sugar
- 4 egg whites, beaten
- 2 cups mashed sweet potatoes
- ¾ cup evaporated skim milk
- 1 tsp. vanilla extract
- ¼ tsp. salt
- ½ tsp. cinnamon
- ½ tsp. nutmeg

Method
1. Preheat oven to 375 degrees.
2. Add egg whites and sugar; add sweet potatoes and mix well.
3. Stir in milk, vanilla, cinnamon, nutmeg and salt, making sure all ingredients are thoroughly mixed.
4. Pour into a greased (non-fat) glass pie plate.
5. Bake for 40 minutes or until knife inserted comes out clean.

Yield: - 4 oz. 8 servings

Nutritional Information
Calories	143
Protein	2.75 grams
Fat	0 grams
Carbs	33 grams

DESSERTS

PUMPKIN PUDDING PIE

Ingredients
- 1 30 oz. can of pumpkin pie mix
- ½ cup of egg substitute or egg whites
- 1 cup evaporated skim milk
- 2 9-inch pie pans

Method
1. Mix pumpkin pie mix, evaporated milk and egg substitute in large bowl.
2. Pour into pie shells.
3. Bake in preheated 425 degree oven for 15 minutes.
4. Reduce temperature to 350 degrees and bake another 50-60 minutes or until knife inserted in center comes out clean.
5. Cool for 2 hours or refrigerate.
6. Serve plain or with fat-free whipped topping (15 calories for 2 tablespoons).

Yield: 12—3.5 oz. servings

Nutritional Information
Calories	97
Protein	3.2 grams
Fat	.4 grams
Carbs	20 grams

OATMEAL COOKIES

Ingredients
- ¾ cup silken tofu
- 1½ cups brown sugar
- ¼ cup apple butter
- ¼ cup egg substitute
- 1 tsp. vanilla
- 1½ cups flour
- 1 tsp. baking soda
- 1 tsp. cinnamon
- ½ tsp. salt
- 3 cups oatmeal
- 1 cup raisins

Method
1. Preheat oven to 350 degrees.
2. Combine silken tofu, brown sugar, apple butter, egg substitute and vanilla in a food processor and mix until well blended.
3. Mix flour, soda, cinnamon and salt in a separate bowl and stir until evenly blended.
4. Slowly stir the tofu mixture into the dry ingredients.
5. When dry mix is moistened, add oats and raisins and continue to stir until oats and raisins are blended into mix.
6. Spray cookie sheets with a non-fat cooking spray and place tablespoon size balls of dough onto sheet.
7. Flatten with spoon and bake for 30–35 minutes.

Yield: 24 cookies (2 cookies per serving)

Nutritional Information
Calories   97
Protein   3 grams
Fat   1.8 grams
Carbs   17 grams

FUDGY BROWNIES

Ingredients
- 1 13.7 oz box of fat-free brownie mix
- ⅔ cup of fat-free vanilla yogurt

Method
1. Preheat oven to 350 degrees.
2. Lightly spray an 8-inch square metal baking pan with cooking spray, wiping off any excess.
3. Pour contents of a box of brownie mix in a medium bowl.
4. Stir in the vanilla yogurt. The batter will be very thick, but keep stirring until all of the powder is combined with the yogurt until it all seems moistened.
5. Spread the mixture into the pan evenly.

6. Bake for 30-35 minutes.

Yield: 12 brownies

Nutritional Information
Calories	110
Protein	2 grams
Fat	0 grams
Carbs	24 grams

REFERENCES

CHAPTER 1:
Nurture Your Own Weight Controller-Athlete

Kelly, K.P., and Kirschenbaum, D.S. (2010). The promise of immersion treatment for obese children and adolescents in 2009: A review. *Obesity and Weight Management, 6,* 35-38.

Kelly, K.P., and Kirschenbaum, D.S. (2011). Immersion treatment for childhood and adolescent obesity: The first review of a promising intervention. *Obesity Reviews, 12,* 37-49.

Kirschenbaum, D. S. (1997). *Mind matters: 7 steps to smarter sport performance.* Carmel, IN: Cooper Publishing Group.

Kirschenbaum, D.S. (2010). Expert recommendations for the treatment of childhood and adolescent obesity: Advantages of the seven step model and immersion treatment. *Journal of Sport Psychology in Action, 1,* 66-75.

Kirschenbaum, D.S., Craig, R., Tjelmeland, L. (2007). *The Sierras weight-loss solution for teens and kids.* NY: Avery. P.169

Kirschenbaum, D.S. (2010). Weight loss camps in the US and the Immersion-to-Lifestyle Change model. *Childhood Obesity, 6,* 318-323.

Kirschenbaum, D.S. (2011). *The Wellspring Weight Loss Plan.* Dallas, TX: BenBella Books.

Kirschenbaum, D.S., Craig, R.D., Kelly, K.P., and Germann, J.N. (2007). Immersion programs for treating pediatric obesity: Follow-up evaluations of Wellspring Camps and Academy of the Sierras—A boarding school for overweight teenagers. *Obesity Management, 3,* 261-266.

CHAPTER 2:
Food Addict: An Unfortunate View of Weight Controllers

American Psychiatric Association (1994). *Diagnostic and statistical manual of mental disorders, Fourth Edition. Text Revision (DSMIV-TR).* Washington, DC: American PsychiatricAssociation.

Barry, C.L. (2012). Public attitudes about addiction as a cause of obesity. In Brownell, K.D., and Gold, M.S. (2012). *Food and addiction: A comprehensive handbook* (pp. 273-280). NY: Oxford.

Brown, P.J. (1993). Cultural perspectives on the etiology and treatment of obesity. In A.J. Stunkard and T.A. Wadden (Eds.) *Obesity: Theory and Therapy, Second Edition* (pp. 179-193). NY: Research Press.

Brownell, K.D., and Gold, M.S. (2012). (Eds.) *Food and addiction: A comprehensive handbook.* NY: Oxford.

Brownell, K.D., and Gold, M.S. (2012). Food and addiction: Scientific, social, legal, and legislative implications. In Brownell, K.D., and Gold, M.S. (2012). *Food and addiction: A comprehensive handbook* (pp. 439-446). NY: Oxford.

Burmeister, J.M. Hinman, N., Hoffmann, D.A., & Carels, R.A. (2013). Food addiction in adults seeking weight loss treatment: Implications for psychosocial health and weight loss. *Appetite*, 60, 103-110.

Fisher, J. D., and Farina, A. (1979). Consequences of beliefs about the nature of mental disorders. *Journal of Abnormal Psychology*, 88, 320-327.

Fitzgibbon, M.L., Stolley, M.R., and Kirschenbaum, D.S. (1993). Obese people who seek treatment have different characteristics than those who do not seek treatment. *Health Psychology*, 12, 342-345.

Gearhart, A.N. and Corbin, W.R. (2012).Food addiction and diagnostic criteria for dependence. In Brownell, K.D., and Gold, M.S. (2012). *Food and addiction: A comprehensive handbook* (pp. 281-284). NY: Oxford.

Greenfield, S.F., and Crisafulli, M.A. (2012). Co-occurring addiction and psychiatric disorders. In Brownell, K.D., and Gold, M.S. (2012). *Food and addiction: A comprehensive handbook* (pp. 47-52). NY: Oxford.

Haddock, C.K., and Poston, W.S.C. (2000). Food as a drug: Conclusions. In Poston, W.S.C. and Haddock, C.K. (2000). (Eds.). *Food as a drug* (141-146). Binghamton, NY: Haworth.

Hudson, J.I., Hiripi, E., Pope, H.G., and Kessler, R.C. (2007). The prevalence and correlates of eating disorders in the NCS replication. *Biological Psychiatry*, 61, 348-358.

Kessler, R.C., Berglund, P.A., Demler, O., Jin, R., and Walters, E.E. (2005). Lifetime prevalence and age-of-onset distributions of DSM-IV disorders in the National Comorbidity Survey Replication (NCS-R). *Archives of General Psychiatry, 62*, 593-602.

Kirkova, D. (2013). "How cravings for food can be as bad as drugs: Food addicts get high after their 'hit' and feel judged like junkie," *Daily Mail*, http://www.dailymail.co.uk/health/article2397942/How-cravings-food-bad-drugs-Food-addicts-high-hit.html.

Kobasa, S. C. (1979). Stressful life events, personality, and health: An inquiry into hardiness. *Journal of Personality and Social Psychology, 37*, 1-11

Koob, G.F. Animals models of drug addiction. In Brownell, K.D., and Gold, M.S. (2012). *Food and addiction: A comprehensive handbook*. NY: Oxford, 3-13.

Lent, M.R., Eichen, D.M., Goldbacher, E., Wadden, T.A., & Foster, G.D. (2014). Relationship of food addiction to weight loss and attriction during obesity treatment. Obesity, 22, 52-55.

Peterson, C. (2000). The future of optimism. *American Psychologist, 55*, 44-55.

Popkin, B.M. (2012). The changing face of global diet and nutrition. In Brownell, K.D., and Gold, M.S. (2012). *Food and addiction: A comprehensive handbook* (pp. 69-80). NY: Oxford.

Poston, W.S.C. and Haddock, C.K. (2000). (Eds.). *Food as a drug*. Binghamton, NY: Haworth.

Scheier, M. F., and Carver, C. S. (1992). Effects of optimism on psychological and physical well-being: Theoretical overview and empirical update. *Cognitive Therapy and Research, 16*, 201–228.

Thaxton, L. (1982). Physiological and psychological effects of short-term exercise addiction on habitual runners. *Journal of Sport Psychology, 4*, 73-80.

CHAPTER 3:
Implications for Weight Controller-Athletes

Baumeister, R. F. (1984). Choking under pressure: Self-consciousness and paradoxical effects of incentives on skillful performance. *Journal of Personality and Social Psychology, 46*, 610-620.

Bloom, B.S. (1985). (Ed.) *Developing talents in young people*. NY: Ballantine Books.

Bruce, L., Farrow, D., and Raynor, A. (2013). Performance milestones in the development of expertise: Are they critical? *Journal of Applied Sport Psychology, 25,* 281-297.

Burton, D. (1989). Winning isn't everything: The impact of performance goals on collegiate swimmers' cognitions and performance. *The Sport Psychologist, 32,*105–132.

Cohn, P.J. (1991). An exploratory study on peak performance in golf. *The Sport Psychologist, 5,* 1-14.

Duda, J.L. (1988). The relationship between goal perspectives, persistence, and intensity among recreational sport participants. *Leisure Sciences, 10,* 95-106.

Ericsson, K.A., and Charness, N. (1994). Expert performance: Its structure and acquisition. *American Psychologist, 49,* 725-747.

Ericsson, K.A., Krampe, R.T., and Tesch-Romar, C. (1993). The role of deliberate practice in the acquisition of expert performance. *Psychological Review, 100,* 363-406.

Fischman, M.G., and Oxendine, J.B. (1993). Motor skill learning for effective coaching and performance. In J.M. Williams (Ed.), *Applied sport psychology: Personal growth to peak performance* (11-24). Mountain View, CA: Mayfield.

Gardner, H. (1973). *The arts and human development.* NY: Wiley.

Garfield, C. A., and Bennett, H.Z. (1984). Mental training techniques of the world's greatest athletes. Los Angeles, CA: J.P. Tarcher. *Golf World,* October 25, 1996.

Jackson, S.A., and Roberts, G.C. (1992). Positive performance states of athletes: Toward a conceptual understanding of peak performance. *The Sport Psychologist, 6,* 156-171.

Kirschenbaum, D.S. (1997). *Mind matters: 7 steps to smarter sport performance.* Carmel, IN: Cooper Publishing Group.

Kirschenbaum, D.S., Fitzgibbon, M.L., Martino, S., Conviser, J.H., Rosendahl, E.H., and Laatsch, L. (1992). Stages of change in successful weight control: A clinically derived model. *Behavior Therapy, 23,* 623-635.

Loehr, J.E. (1984). How to overcome stress and play at your peak all the time. *Tennis, March,* 66-76.

Ravissa, K. (1984). Qualities of the peak experience in sport. In J.M. Silva and R.S. Weinberg (Eds.). *Psychological foundations of sport* (452-462). Champaign, IL: Human Kinetics.

Weinberg, R.S. (1988). *The mental advantage.* Champaign, IL: Leisure Press.

Wing, R.R., and Hill, J.O. (2001). Successful weight loss maintenance. *Annual Review of Nutrition, 21,* 323-341.

Young, E. (1858). *The poetical works of Edward Young.* London: Bell & Daldy.

CHAPTER 4:
Becoming Overweight: Causes and Fixes

Barnard, N.D., Akhtar, A., and Nicholson, A. (1995). Factors that facilitate compliance to lower fat intake. *Archives of Family Medicine, 4,* 153-158.

Bessesen, D.H., Rupp, C.L., and Eckel, R.H. (1995). Dietary fat is shunted away from oxidation, toward storage in obese Zucker rats. *Obesity Research, 3,* 179-189.

Blass, E. (1989). Opioids, sweets, and a mechanism for positive affect: Broad motivational implications. In J. Dobbing (Ed.) *Sweetness.* NY: Springer-Verlag.

Blundell, J.E., Burley, V.J., Cotton, J.R., and Lawton, C.L. (1993). Dietary fat in the control of energy intake: Evaluating the effects of fat on meal size and postmeal satiety. *American Journal of Clinical Nutrition, 57,* 772S-778S.

Boozer, C.N., Brasseur, A., and Atkinson, R.L. (1993). Dietary fat affects weight loss and adiposity during energy restriction in rats. *American Journal of Clinical Nutrition, 58,* 846-852.

Bouchard, C., Tremblay, A., and Depres, J. (1990). The response to long-term overfeeding in identical twins. *New England Journal of Medicine, 322,* 1477-1482.

Braet, C. (2006). Patient characteristics as predictors of weight loss after an obesity treatment for children. *Obesity, 14,* 148-155.

Brownell, K.D. and Horgen, K.B. (2004). *Food fight.* Chicago: Contemporary Books.

Critser, G. (2004). *Fat Land.* Boston: Mariner.

Dietz, W. H., and Robinson, T.N. (2005). Overweight children and adolescents. *New England Journal of Medicine, 352,* 2100-2109.

Dobbing, J. (Ed.). (1987). *Sweetness.* NY: Springer-Verlag.

Epstein, L.H., Valoski, A., Wing, R.R., and McCurley, J. (1994). Ten-year outcomes of behavioral family-based treatment for childhood obesity. *Health Psychology, 13,* 373-383.

Geiselman, P.J., and Novin, D. (1982). The role of carbohydrates in appetite, hunger and obesity. *Appetite, 3*, 203-223.

Gosling, S.D., Rentfrow, P.J., and Swann, W.B. (2003). A very brief measure of the Big-Five personality domains. *Journal of Research in Personality, 37*, 504-528.

Hampson, S.E., Edmonds, G.W., Goldberg, L.R., Dubanoski, J.P., and Hillier, T.A. (2013). Childhood conscientiousness relates to objectively measured adult physical health four decades later. *Health Psychology, 32*, 925-928.

Hartigan, K.J., Baker-Strauch, D., and Morris, G.W. (1982). Perceptions of the causes of obesity and responsiveness to treatment. *Journal of Counseling Psychology, 29*, 478-485.

Hedley, A.A. et al. (2004). Prevalence of overweight and obesity among US children, adolescents, and adults, 1999-2002. *Journal of the American Medical Association, 291*, 2847-2850.

Heska, S., Anderson, J.W., Atkinson, R.L., Greenway, F.L., Hill, J.O., Phinney, S.D., and Pi-Sunyer, F.X. (2003). Weight loss with self-help compared with a structured commercial program: A randomized trial. *Journal of the American Medical Association, 289*, 1792-1798.

Hill, J.O., Drougas, H., and Peters, J.C. (1993). Obesity treatment: Can diet composition play a role? *Annals of Internal Medicine, 119*, 694-697.

Jeffery, R.W., Hellerstedt, W.L., French, S.A. and Baxter, J.E. (1995). A randomized trial of counseling for fat restriction versus calorie restriction in the treatment of obesity. *International Journal of Obesity, 19*, 132-137.

Jeffery, R.W., Wing, R.R., and Mayer, R.R. (1998). Are smaller weight losses or more achievable weight loss goals better in the long term for obese patients? *Journal of Consulting and Clinical Psychology, 66*, 641-645.

Kelly, K.P., and Kirschenbaum, D.S. (2011). Immersion treatment for childhood and adolescent obesity: The first review of a promising intervention. *Obesity Reviews, 12*, 37-49.

Kirschenbaum, D.S. (2010). Weight loss camps in the US and the Immersion-to-Lifestyle Change model. *Childhood Obesity, 6*, 318-323.

Kirschenbaum, D.S., Fitzgibbon, M.L., Martino, S., Conviser, J.H., Rosendahl, E.H., and Laatsch, L. (1992). Stages of change in successful weight control: A clinically derived model. *Behavior Therapy, 23*, 623-635.

Kirschenbaum, D.S., and Gierut, K.J. (2013). Treatment of childhood and adolescent obesity: An integrative review of recent recommendations from five expert groups. *Journal of Consulting and Clinical Psychology, 81*, 347-360.

Kramer, F.M., Jeffery, R.W., Forster, J.L., and Snell, M.K. (1989). Long-term follow-up of behavioral treatment for obesity: Patterns of weight regain among men and women. *International Journal of Obesity, 13*, 123-136.

Lang, Peter J. (1995). The emotion probe: Studies of motivation and attention. *American Psychologist,50*, 372-385.

Liebman, B. (2004). Fat: More than just a lump of lard. *Nutrition Action Health Letter, 31*, 1-6.

McAdams, D.P., and Pals, J.L. (2006). A new big five : Fundamental principles for an integrative science of personality. *American Psychologist, 61*, 204-217.

Nader, P.R. et al. (2006). Identifying risk for obesity in early childhood. *Pediatrics, 118*, e594-e601.

Ogden, C.L. et al. (2002). Prevalence and trends in overweight among US children and adolescents, 199-2000. *Journal of the American Medical Association, 288*, 1728-1732.

Powell, L.H., Calvin, J.E., and Calvin, J.E. (2007). Effective obesity treatments. *American Psychologist, 62*, 234-246.

Ravussin, E., and Swinburn, B.A. (1993). Energy metabolism. In A.J. Stunkard and T.A. Wadden (Eds.) *Obesity: Theory and Therapy, Second Edition*. New York: Raven Press.

Sims, E.Z.H., Danforth, E., et al. (1973). Endocrine and metabolic effects of experimental obesity in man. *Recent Progress in Hormone Research, 29*, 457-487.

Schwimmer, J.B., Burwinkle, T.M., and Varni, J.W. (2003). Health-related quality of life of severely obese children and adolescents. *Journal of the American Medical Association, 289*, 1813-1819.

Skelton, J. A., Goff, D. C., Ip, E., and Beech, B. M. (2011). Attrition in a multidisciplinary Pediatric weight management clinic. *Childhood Obesity, 7*, 185–193.

Stice, E., Shaw, H., and Marti, C.N. (2006). A meta-analytic review of obesity prevention programs for children and adolescents: The skinny on interventions that work. *Psychological Bulletin, 132*(5), 667-691.

Stunkard, A.J. (1958). The management of obesity. *New York State Journal of Medicine, 58*, 79-87.

Wadden, T.A. (1993). Treatment of obesity by moderate and severe caloric restriction: Results of clinical research trials. *Annals of Internal Medicine, 119,* 688-693

Wadden, T.A. et al. (1997). Lifestyle modification in the pharmacologic treatment of obesity: A pilot investigation of a potential primary care approach. *Obesity Research, 5,* 218-226.

Wadden, T.A. and A. J. Stunkard (2002).(Eds.) *Handbook of Obesity Treatment.* New York: Guilford Press.

Wang, Y., and Lobstein, T. (2006).Worldwide trends in childhood and adolescent obesity. *International Journal of Pediatric Obesity, 1,* 11-25.

CHAPTER 5:
Step 1: Understand Your Body's Resistance to Weight Loss

Barnard, N.D., Akhtar, A., and Nicholson, A. (1995). Factors that facilitate compliance to lower fat intake. *Archives of Family Medicine, 4,*153-158.

Bessesen, D.H., Rupp, C.L., and Eckel, R.H. (1995). Dietary fat is shunted away from oxidation, toward storage in obese Zucker rats. *Obesity Research, 3,*179-189.

Blass, E. (1989). Opioids, sweets, and a mechanism for positive affect: Broad motivational implications. In J. Dobbing (Ed.) *Sweetness.* NY: Springer-Verlag.

Blundell, J.E., Burley, V.J., Cotton, J.R., and Lawton, C.L. (1993). Dietary fat in the control of energy intake: Evaluating the effects of fat on meal size and postmeal satiety. *American Journal of Clinical Nutrition, 57,* 772S-778S.

Boozer, C.N., Brasseur, A., and Atkinson, R.L. (1993). Dietary fat affects weight loss and adiposity during energy restriction in rats. *American Journal of Clinical Nutrition, 58,* 846-852.

Dobbing, J. (Ed.). (1987). *Sweetness.* NY: Springer-Verlag.

Epstein, L.H., Valoski, A., Wing, R.R., and McCurley, J. (1994). Ten-year outcomes of behavioral family-based treatment for childhood obesity. *Health Psychology, 13,* 373-383.

Geiselman, P.J., and Novin, D. (1982). The role of carbohydrates in appetite, hunger and obesity. *Appetite, 3,* 203-223.

Hartigan, K.J., Baker-Strauch, D., and Morris, G.W. (1982). Perceptions of the causes of obesity and responsiveness to treatment. *Journal of Counseling Psychology, 29,* 478-485.

Hill, J.O., Drougas, H., and Peters, J.C. (1993). Obesity treatment: Can diet composition play a role? *Annals of Internal Medicine, 119,* 694-697.

Jeffery, R.W., Hellerstedt, W.L., French, S.A. and Baxter, J.E. (1995). A randomized trial of counseling for fat restriction versus calorie restriction in the treatment of obesity. *International Journal of Obesity, 19,* 132-137.

Jeffery, R.W., Wing, R.R., and Mayer, R.R. (1998). Are smaller weight losses or more achievable weight loss goals better in the long term for obese patients? *Journal of Consulting and Clinical Psychology, 66,* 641-645.

Johnson, W.G., and Wilman, H.E. (1983). Influence of external and covert food stimuli on insulin secretion in obese and normal persons. *Behavioral Neuroscience, 97,* 1025-1028.

Kirschenbaum, D.S. et al. (1992). Stages of change in successful weight control: A clinically derived model. *Behavior Therapy, 23,* 623-635.

Kramer, F.M., Jeffery, R.W., Forster, J.L., and Snell, M.K. (1989). Long-term follow-up of behavioral treatment for obesity: Patterns of weight regain among men and women. *International Journal of Obesity, 13,* 123-136.

Liebman, B. (2004). Fat: More than just a lump of lard. *Nutrition Action Health Letter, 31,* 1-6.

Ravussin, E., and Swinburn, B.A. (1993). Energy metabolism. In A.J. Stunkard and T.A. Wadden (Eds.) *Obesity: Theory and Therapy, Second Edition.* New York: Raven Press.

Sims, E.Z.H., Danforth, E., et al. (1973). Endocrine and metabolic effects of experimental obesity in man. *Recent Progress in Hormone Research, 29,* 457-487.

Staff Writer (1996). Weight-loss news that's easy to stomach. *Tufts University Diet and Nutrition Letter, 14,* 1.

Stunkard, A.J. (1958). The management of obesity. *New York State Journal of Medicine, 58,* 79-87.

Wadden, T.A. (1993). Treatment of obesity by moderate and severe caloric restriction: Results of clinical research trials. *Annals of Internal Medicine, 119,* 688-693.

Wadden, T.A. et al. (1997). Lifestyle modification in the pharmacologic treatment of obesity: A pilot investigation of a potential primary care approach. *Obesity Research, 5,* 218-226.

CHAPTER 6:
Step 2: Create a Powerful Commitment to Succeed

Hubbel, M.A., Duncan, B.L., and Miller, S.D. (1999). (Eds.). *The heart and soul of change: What works in therapy.* Washington, D.C.: American Psychological Association.

Janis, I.L., and Mann, L. (1977). *Decision making: A psychological analysis of conflict, choice, and commitment.* NY: The Free Press.

Kirsch, I. (1990). *Changing expectations: A key to effective psychotherapy.* Pacific Grove, CA: Brooks/Cole.

Kirschenbaum, D.S., Fitzgibbon, M.L., Martino, S., Conviser, J.H., Rosendahl, E.H., and Laatsch, L. (1992). Stages of change in successful weight control: A clinically derived model. *Behavior Therapy, 23,* 623-635.

Meichenbaum, D., and Turk, D.C. (1987). *Facilitating treatment adherence: A practitioner's guidebook.* New York: Plenum.

Nelson, L.R., and Furst, M.L. (1972). An objective study of the effects of expectation on competitive performance. *Journal of Psychology, 81,* 69-72.

Shapiro, A.K. (1978). Placebo effects in medicine, psychotherapy, and psychoanalysis. In A.P. Bergin and S.L. Garfield (1973).(Eds.). *Handbook of Psychotherapy and Behavior Change: An empirical analysis.* New York: John Wiley.

Vincent, P. (1971). Factors influencing patient noncompliance: A theoretical approach. *Nursing Research, 20,* 509-516.

Wang, S.S., Houshyar, S. and Prinstein, M.J. (2006). Adolescent girls' and boys' weight-related health behaviors and cognitions: Associations with reputation- and preference-based peer status. *Health Psychology, 25,* 658-663.

Wadden, T. A., Womble, L.G., Stunkard, A.J., and Anderson, D.A. (2002). Psychosocial consequences of obesity and weight loss. In T.A. Wadden and A. J. Stunkard (Eds.) *Handbook of Obesity Treatment.* New York: Guilford Press.

CHAPTER 7:
Step 3: Manage Food to Lose Weight Most Comfortably

Agatston, A. (2003). *The South Beach diet: The delicious, doctor-designed, foolproof plan for fast and healthy weight loss.* Emmaus, PA: Rodale Press.

References

Alfieri, M.A.H, Pomerleau, J., Grace, D.M., and Anderson, L. (1995). Fiber intake of normal weight, moderately obese and severely obese subjects. *Obesity Research, 3,* 541-547.

"Are you eating right? Most of us think so, our poll finds," *Consumer Reports News*: January 06, 2011 http://www.consumerreports.org/cro/news/2011/01/are-you-eating-right-most-of-us-think-so-our-poll-finds/index.htm

Atkins, R.C. (1998). *Dr. Atkins' New diet revolution*. New York, NY: Avon Books.

Barnard, N.D., Akhtar, A., and Nicholson, A. (1995). Factors that facilitate compliance to lower fat intake. *Archives of Family Medicine, 4,* 153-158.

Bessesen, D.H., Rupp, C.L., and Eckel, R.H. (1995). Dietary fat is shunted away from oxidation, toward storage in obese Zucker rats. *Obesity Research, 3,*179-189.

Boozer, C.N., Brasseur, A., and Atkinson, R.L. (1993). Dietary fat affects weight loss and adiposity during energy restriction in rats. *American Journal of Clinical Nutrition, 58,* 846-852.

Borushek, A. (2012). *The Calorie King calorie fat and carbohydrate counter*. Costa Mesa, CA: Family Health Publications.

Brownell, K.D. and Horgen, K.B. (2004). *Food fight*. Chicago: Contemporary Books.

Campbell, T.C. with Campbell, T.M. (2005). *The China Study: Startling implications for diet, weight loss, and long-term health*. Dallas, TX: BenBella Books.

Centers for Disease Control Press Release 2/5/2004: Calorie consumption on the rise in United States, particularly among women. http://www.cdc.gov/nchs/pressroom/04news/calorie. htm.

CSPI (2011). *Ten super foods for better health*. Washington, DC: CSPI. See www.cspinet.org for more details and http://www.cspinet.org/nah/10foods_us.pdf.

Critser, G. (2004). *Fat Land*. Boston: Mariner.

Fleming, R.M. (2002). The effect of high-, moderate-, and low-fat diets on weight loss and cardiovascular disease risk factors. *Preventive Cardiology, 5,* 110-118.

Harris, J.K., French, S.A., Jeffery, R.W., McGovern, P., and Wing, R.R. (1994). Dietary and physical activity correlates of long-term weight loss. *Obesity Research, 2,* 307-313.

Kirschenbaum, D.S. (2000). *The 9 truths about weight loss*. NY: Holt.

Kirschenbaum, D.S. (2005). Very low-fat diets are much better than low-carbohydrate diets: A position paper based on science. *Patient Care, 39,* 47-55.

Mann, T., Tomiyana, A.J. et al. (2007). Medicare's search for effective obesity treatments: Diets are not the answer. *American Psychologist, 62,* 220-233.

Rozin, P., Ashmore, M., and Markwith, M. (1996). Lay conceptions of nutrition: Dose insensitivity, categorical thinking, contagion, and the monotonic mind. *Health Psychology, 15,* 438-447.

Sears, B. and Lawren, B. (1995).*The zone: A dietary road map to lose weight permanently, reset your genetic code, prevent disease, achieve maximum physical performance.* New York: HarperCollins.

Shick, S.M., Wing, R.E., Klem, M.L., McGuire, M.T., Hill, J.O., and Seagle, H. (1998). Persons successful at long-term weight loss and maintenance continue to consume a low-energy, low-fat diet. *Journal of the American Dietetic Association, 98,* 408-413.

Stice, E. (1998). Prospective relation of dieting behaviors to weight change in a community sample of adolescents. *Behavior Therapy, 29,* 277-297.

Stubbs, R.J. (1995). Macronutrient effects on appetite. *International Journal of Obesity and Related Metabolic Disorders, 19 (sup.5),* S11-S19.

Van Horn, L., and Kavey, R.E. (1997). Diet and cardiovascular disease prevention: What works? *Annals of Behavioral Medicine, 19,* 197-212.

Wadden, T.A., and Osei, S. (2002). The treatment of obesity: An overview. In T.A.Wadden and A.J. Stunkard (Eds.) *Handbook of obesity treatment.* New York: Guilford Press, 229-248.

Weigle, D.S., Cummings, D.E., et al. (2003). Roles of leptin and ghrelin in the loss of body weight caused by a low-fat, high carbohydrate diet. *Journal of Clinical and Endocrinological Metabolism, 88,* 1577-1586.

World Cancer Research Fund / American Institute for Cancer Research (2007). *Food, nutrition, physical activity, and the prevention of cancer: A global perspective.* Washington DC: American Institute for Cancer Research.

CHAPTER 8:
Step 4: Use Movement to Level the Playing Field

Andersen, R.E., Wadden, T.A., Bartlett, S.J., Zemel, B., Verde, T.J., and Franckowiak, S.C (1999). Effects of lifestyle activity vs structured aerobic exercise in obese women: A randomized trial. *Journal of the American Medical Association, 281,*335-340.

Baechle, T.R., and Groves, B.R. (1992). *Weight training: Steps to success.* Champaign, IL: Leisure Press.

Blair, S.N. (1991). *Living with exercise.* Dallas, TX: American Health Publishing Co.

Blair, S.N. (1991). Weight loss through physical activity. *Weight Control Digest, 1,* 17, 20-24.

Carpenter, R.A. (2004). Getting in step with counters. *Weight Management Newsletter of the American Dietetic Association. 1,* 1-2.

Curless, M.R. (1992). Only the fit stay young. *Self,* September, pp. 180-181.

Dishman, R.K. (Ed.). (1988). *Exercise adherence: Its impact on public health.* Champaign, IL: Human Kinetics Publishers.

Donahoe, C.P., Jr., Lin, D.H., Kirschenbaum, D.S., and Keesey, R.E. (1984). Metabolic consequences of dieting and exercise in the treatment of obesity. *Journal of Consulting and Clinical Psychology, 52,* 827-836.

Galvin, J. (1991). *The exercise habit: Your personal road map to developing a lifelong exercise commitment.* Champaign, IL: Human Kinetics Publishers.

Heil, J. (1993). *Psychology of sport injury.* Champaign, IL: Human Kinetics Publishers.

Kendzierski, D., and Johnson, W. (1993). Excuses, excuses, excuses: A cognitive behavioral approach to exercise implementation. *Journal of Sport and Exercise Psychology, 15,* 207-219.

Kirschenbaum, D.S. (1998). *Mind matters: Seven steps to smarter sport performance.* Carmel, Indiana: Cooper Publishing Group.

Kusinitz, I., Fin, M., and Editors of Consumer Reports Books. (1983). *Physical fitness for practically everybody: The consumer's union report on exercise.* Mount Vernon: NY: Consumers Union.

Latella, F.S., Conkling, W., and Editors of Consumers Reports Books. (1989). *Get in shape stay in shape.* NY: Consumer Reports Books.

Rippe, J.M., and Amend, P. (1992). *The exercise exchange program.* NY: Simon and Schuster.

Vickery, S. and Moffat, M. (1999).*The American Physical Therapy Association book of body repair and maintenance.* NY: Owl Books.

CHAPTER 9:
Step 5: Develop an Athlete's Healthy Obsession

Baker, R.C., and Kirschenbaum, D.S. (1993). Self-monitoring may be necessary for successful weight control. *Behavior Therapy, 24,* 377-394.

Baker, R.C., and Kirschenbaum, D.S. (1998). Weight control during the holidays: Highly consistent self-monitoring as a potentially useful coping mechanism. *Health Psychology, 17,* 367-370.

Barnard, N.D., Akhtar, A., and Nicholson, A. (1995). Factors that facilitate compliance to lower fat intake. *Archives of Family Medicine, 4,* 153-158.

Braet, C. and Van Winckel, M. (2000). Long-term follow-up of a cognitive behavioral treatment program for obese children. *Behavior Therapy, 31,* 55-74.

Baumeister, R.F., Heatherton, T.F., and Tice, D.M. (1994). *Losing control: How and why people fail at self-regulation.* San Diego, CA: Academic Press.

Bessesen, D.H., Rupp, C.L., and Eckel, R.H. (1995). Dietary fat is shunted away from oxidation, toward storage in obese Zucker rats. *Obesity Research, 3,* 179-189.

Boozer, C.N., Brasseur, A., and Atkinson, R.L. (1993). Dietary fat affects weight loss and adiposity during energy restriction in rats. *American Journal of Clinical Nutrition, 58,* 846-852.

Boutelle, K.N., and Kirschenbaum, D.S. (1998). Further support for consistent self-monitoring as a vital component of successful weight control. *Obesity Research, 6,* 219-224.

Boutelle, K.N., Kirschenbaum, D.S., Baker, R.C., and Mitchell, M.E. (1999). How can obese weight controllers minimize weight gain during the high-risk holiday season? By self-monitoring very consistently. *Health Psychology, 18,* 364-368.

Calvin Coolidge Memorial Foundation, *Coolidge Resources,* http://www.calvin-coolidge.org/quotations-p.html.

Campbell, T.C. with Campbell, T.M. (2005). *The China Study: Startling implications for diet, weight loss, and long-term health.* Dallas, TX: BenBella Books.

Carver, C.S., and Scheier, M.F. (1990). Origins and functions of positive and negative affect: A control-process view. *Psychological Review, 97,* 19-35.

Ericsson, K.A., and Charness, N. (1994). Expert performance: Its structure and acquisition. *American Psychologist, 49,* 725-747.

Dobbing, J. (Ed.). (1987). *Sweetness.* NY: Springer-Verlag Kirschenbaum, D.S. (1987). Self-regulatory failure: A review with clinical implications. *Clinical Psychology Review, 7,* 77-104.

Gately, P.J., Cooke, C.B., Butterly, R.J., Mackreth, P., and Carroll, S. (2000). The effects of a children's summer camp programme on weight loss, with a 10 month follow-up. *International Journal of Obesity, 24,* 1445-1453.

Gierut, K.J., and Kirschenbaum, D.S. (2013). "I see inspiration everywhere": Potential keys to nurturing healthy obsessions by very successful adolescent weight controllers. *Childhood Obesity.*

Gierut, K.J., Pecora, K.M., and Kirschenbaum, D.S. (2012). Highly successful weight control by formerly obese adolescents: A qualitative test of the healthy obsession model. *Childhood Obesity, 8,* 455-465.

Geiselman, P.J., and Novin, D. (1982). The role of carbohydrates in appetite, hunger and obesity. *Appetite, 3,* 203-223.

Harris, J.K., French, S.A., Jeffery, R.W., McGovern, P., and Wing, R.R. (1994). Dietary and physical activity correlates of long-term weight loss. *Obesity Research, 2,* 307-313.

Hensen, C.J., Stevens, L.C., and Coast, J.R. (2001). Exercise duration and mood state: How much is enough to feel better? *Health Psychology, 20,* 267-275.

Hill, J.O., Drouglas, H., and Peters, J.C. (1993). Obesity treatment: Can diet composition play a role? *Annals of Internal Medicine, 119,* 694-697.

Hume, K.M., Martin, G.L., Gonzalez, P., Kracklen, C., and Genthon, S. (1985). A self-monitoring feedback package for improving freestyle figure skating practice. *Journal of Sport Psychology, 7,* 138-166.

Israel, A.C., and Shapiro, L.S. (1985). Behavior problems of obese children enrolling in a weight reduction program. *Cognitive Therapy and Research, 6,* 451-460.

Jeffery, R.W., Hellerstedt, W.L., French, S.A. and Baxter, J.E. (1995). A randomized trial of counseling for fat restriction versus calorie restriction in the treatment of obesity. *International Journal of Obesity, 19,* 132-137.

Kanfer, F.H., and Karoly, P. (1972). Self-control: A behavioristic excursion into the lion's den. *Behavior Therapy, 3,* 398-416.

Kirschenbaum, D.S. (1987). Self-regulatory failure: A review with clinical implications. *Clinical Psychology Review, 7,* 77-104.

Kirschenbaum, D.S. (1994). *Weight loss through persistence: Making science work for you.* Oakland, CA: New Harbinger.

Kirschenbaum, D.S. (2000). *The 9 truths about weight loss.* NY: Holt.

Kirschenbaum, D.S. (2006) *The healthy obsession program: Smart weight loss instead of low-carb lunacy.* Dallas, TX: BenBella Books,.

Kirschenbaum, D.S. (2011). *The Wellspring Weight Loss Plan.* Dallas, TX: BenBella Books.

Kirschenbaum, D.S., Craig, R.D., Kelly, K.P., and Germann, J.N. (2007). Immersion programs for treating pediatric obesity: Follow-up evaluations of Wellspring Camps and Academy of the Sierras - a therapeutic boarding school. *ObesityManagement, 3*, 261-266.

Kirschenbaum, D.S., Germann, J.N., and Rich, B.H. (2005). Treatment of morbid obesity in low-income minority adolescents: Participant and parental self-monitoring as determinants of initial success. *Obesity Research, 13*, 1527-1529.

Kirschenbaum, D.S., and Karoly, P. (1977). When self-regulation fails: Tests of some preliminary hypotheses. *Journal of Consulting and Clinical Psychology, 45*, 1116-1125.

McGuire, M.T., Wing, R.R., Klem, M.L., Lang, W. and Hill, J.O. (1999). What predicts weight regain in a group of successful weight losers? *Journal of Consulting and Clinical Psychology, 67*, 177-185.

McGuire, M.T., Wing, R.R., Klem, M.L., and Hill, J.O. (1999). Behavioral strategies of individuals who have maintained long-term weight losses. *Obesity Research, 7*, 334-341.

Perri, M.G., Anton, S.D. et al. (2002). Adherence to exercise prescriptions: Effects of prescribing moderate versus higher levels of intensity and frequency. *Health Psychology, 21*, 452-458.

Perri, M.G., Nezu, A.M., and Viegener, B.J. (1992). *Improving the long-term management of obesity: Theory, research and clinical guidelines.* New York: John Wiley.

Schlundt, D.G., Sbrocco, T., and Bell, C. (1989). Identification of high-risk situations in a behavioral weight loss program: Application of the relapse prevention model. *International Journal of Obesity, 13*, 223-234.

Sperduto, W.A., Thompson, H.S., and O'Brien, R.M. (1986). The effect of target behavior monitoring on weight loss and completion rate in a behavior modification program for weight reduction. *Addictive Behaviors, 11*, 337-340.

Stice E.(1998). Prospective relation of dieting behaviors to weight change in a community sample of adolescents. *Behavior Therapy, 29*, 277-297.

Subrahmanyam, K., Kraut, R.E., Greenfield, P.M., and Gross, E. F. (2000). The impact of home computer use on children's activities and development. *Children and Computer Technology, 10*, 123-140.

Weinberg, R.S. (1988). *The mental advantage: Developing your psychological skills in tennis.* Champaign, IL: Leisure Press.

CHAPTER 10:
Step 6: Build a Winning Team around You

Davis, M., Eshelman, E.R. and McKay, M. (1995). *The relaxation and stress reduction workbook* (4thed.). Oakland, CA: New Harbinger Publications, Inc.

Kirschenbaum, D.S. (1997). *Mind matters: 7 steps to smarter sport performance.* Carmel, IN: Cooper Publishing Group.

McKay, M., and Fanning, P. (1993). *Time out from stress.* Oakland, CA: New Harbinger Publications, Inc.

Paine, W.S. (1982) (Ed.). *Job stress and burnout.* Beverly Hills, CA: Sage Publications.

Smith, R.E., Smoll, F.L., and Curtis, B. (1979). Coach effectiveness training: A cognitive-behavioral approach to enhancing relationship skills in youth sport coaches. *Journal of Sport Psychology, 1, 59-75.*

Weinberg, R.S., and Gould, D. (2006). *Foundations of sport and exercise psychology,* Fourth Edition. Champaign, IL: Human Kinetics.

CHAPTER 11:
Step 7: Become Undisturbable

Alberti, R.E., and Emmons, M.L.(1990). *Your perfect right: A guide to assertive living* (6thed.). San Luis Obispo, CA: Impact Publishers.

Barlow, D.H., and Rapee, R.M. (1991). *Mastering stress: A lifestyle approach.* Dallas: American Health Publishing Company.

Bourne, E.J. (1990). *The anxiety and phobia workbook.* Oakland, CA: New Harbinger Publications, Inc.

Burns, D.E. (1989). *The feeling good handbook: Using the new mood therapy in everyday life.* NY: William Morrow and Company.

Cautela, J.R., and Groden, J. (1991). *Relaxation: A comprehensive manual for adults, children, and children with special needs.* Champaign, IL: Research Press.

Davis, M., Eshelman, E.R. and McKay, M. (1995). *The relaxation and stress reduction workbook* (4thed.). Oakland, CA: New Harbinger Publications, Inc.

Ellis, A., and Harper, R.A. (1975). *A new guide to rational living.* Hollywood, CA: Wilshire Book Co.

Grasha, A.F., and Kirschenbaum, D.S. (1986). *Adjustment and competence: Concepts and applications.* Minneapolis: West Publishing Company.

Harp, D., with Feldman, N. (1990). *The new three minute meditator.* Oakland, CA: New Harbinger Publications, Inc.

Holmes, T.H., and Rahe, R.H. (1967). The social readjustment rating scale. *Journal of Psychosomatic Research, 11,* 216.

Kirschenbaum, D.S., and Wittrock, D.A. (1990). Still searching for effective criticism inoculation procedures. *Journal of Applied Sport Psychology, 2,* 175-185.

Marlatt, G.A., and Donovan, D.M. (2005). (Eds.) *Relapse prevention: Maintenance strategies in the treatment of addictive behaviors.* NY: Guildford.

Marks, I.M. (1978). *Living with fear: Understanding and coping with anxiety.* NY: McGraw-Hill.

Meichenbaum, D. (1985). *Stress inoculation training.* NY: Pergamon.

Seligman, M.E.P. (1995). The effectiveness of psychotherapy. *American Psychologist, 50,* 965–974.

Stevens, J.O. (1971). *Awareness: Exploring, experimenting, experiencing.* Moab, Utah: Real People Press.

Thayer, R.E. (1987). Energy, tiredness, and tension effects of a sugar snack versus moderate exercise. *Journal of Personality and Social Psychology, 52,* 119-125.

Tubesing, N.L., and Tubesing, D.H. (1990). *Structured exercises in stress management.* (vols. 1-4). Duluth, MN: Whole Person Press.

Zilberg, N.J., Weiss, D.S., and Horowitz, M.J. (1982). Impact of Event Scale: A Cross-Validation Study. *Journal of Consulting and Clinical Psychology, 50,* 407-414.